Democracy in the Time of Coronavirus

THE RANDY L.

AND MELVIN R. BERLIN

FAMILY LECTURES

Democracy in the Time of Coronavirus

DANIELLE ALLEN

The University of Chicago Press
Chicago and London

The University of Chicago Press gratefully acknowledges
the generous support of the Randy L. and Melvin R. Berlin Family
Endowment toward the publication of this book.

The University of Chicago Press, Chicago 60637
The University of Chicago Press, Ltd., London
© 2022 by Democratic Knowledge, LLC

Published 2022
Printed in the United States of America

31 30 29 28 27 26 25 24 23 22   1 2 3 4 5

ISBN-13: 978-0-226-81560-2 (cloth)
ISBN-13: 978-0-226-81562-6 (paper)
ISBN-13: 978-0-226-81561-9 (e-book)
DOI: https://doi.org/10.7208/chicago/9780226815619.001.0001

Library of Congress Cataloging-in-Publication Data

Names: Allen, Danielle S., 1971–, author.
Title: Democracy in the time of coronavirus / Danielle Allen.
Other titles: Randy L. and Melvin R. Berlin family lectures.
Description: Chicago : University of Chicago Press, 2022. |
Series: Berlin family lectures | Includes bibliographical references and index.
Identifiers: LCCN 2021024484 | ISBN 9780226815602 (cloth) |
ISBN 9780226815626 (paperback) | ISBN 9780226815619 (ebook)
Subjects: LCSH: COVID-19 Pandemic, 2020—Political aspects—United States. |
Democracy—United States. | Crisis management in government—
United States. | United States—Politics and government—2017–.
Classification: LCC RA644.C67 A47 2021 | DDC 362.1962/414—dc23
LC record available at https://lccn.loc.gov/2021024484

♾ This paper meets the requirements of ANSI/NISO Z39.48-1992
(Permanence of Paper).

Dedicated to the more than six hundred thousand Americans dead from COVID-19

Contents

Preface

When the new coronavirus arrived in the United States in January 2020, it hit an economy, society, and constitutional democracy fundamentally unprepared. As the scale of the challenge became clear, the country simply could not deliver what was needed to confront it. There was a solution, one identified by scholars and policy experts as early as the middle of March and publicly disseminated by the middle of April. That solution was a large-scale program of rapid testing of patients, tracing and testing their contacts, and tracing and testing their contacts again in turn. Such testing also needed reinforcement from a culture of adherence to universal precautions such as mask-wearing, hand and bathroom hygiene, and robust practices of infection control. The massive, rapid buildup of such a public health campaign, as well as the necessary infrastructure to support it, would have interrupted transmission of the virus sufficiently to eliminate it even while keeping the economy open. But the country did not have the relevant infrastructure ready to go and was not able to deliver this mobilization.

Just as the 2008 financial crisis exposed blind spots in how countries had thought about integrated markets through the first stages of globalization, within the first two months of 2020, the spread of COVID-19 revealed that the United States had another gaping vulnerability to globalization. Like opaque securities, pandemics proved to be a dangerous feature of globally integrated markets. We learned that, given the modern structure of travel, transportation, and integrated economies, infectious pathogens travel as easily as the Davos elite.

The near-term challenge of January 2020 was identical to our long-term challenge: how to achieve pandemic resilience—the ability of our social and political institutions to process a major exogenous shock yet keep all essential functions operating, while simultaneously protecting lives, livelihoods, and liberties. The urgency of the crisis meant that we needed to deliver the durable infrastructure of resilience in the form of emergency response. But the near-term nature of the crisis situation by no means required that the response to it should consist only of transient initiatives. Emergencies have always provided opportunities for durable innovation.

Look back to antiquity. The Romans' Appian Way, their first major road, was built in 312 BCE as a supply line during the Second Samnite War. A crisis response yielded durable infrastructure. Of course, the same kind of thing happened with penicillin and nuclear power in World War II (Conant 2017; Johnstone-Louis et al. 2020). A crisis will by its nature elicit reactive action of some kind. The question is only whether in its reactions a society lays down a foundation for a better future or expends its energies on changeable, flailing efforts. In our own situation, the effort to find a vaccine to protect against COVID-19 is another good example of an emergency yielding a permanent advance. The Moderna variant uses a technology, synthetic messenger RNA, that has never before been used for vaccine production (Garde and Saltzmann 2020). In all likelihood we will leave this crisis with an important new tool firmly entrenched in the health-care toolkit. We could have and should have done the same with the infrastructure of public health.

In this book, I hope to lay the foundation for a renewed social contract capable of delivering pandemic resilience—and, more generally, both justice and health for our constitutional democracy. I hope to offer a durable breakthrough in the form of a fresh vision of the public good.

What exactly is a social contract? A social contract is the set of rights and mutual responsibilities that we have among ourselves as citizens in a constitutional democracy. A social contract is both what's asked of us as participants in a constitutional democracy and all that is made possible for us by virtue of our participation in that constitutional democracy. What's asked of us and what we receive establish relations of reciprocity within the citizenry. This book seeks to reset that relationship for a healthy and just future.

The pandemic revealed that our social contract is fundamentally broken. Our society includes people who are being asked to follow the law and to pay taxes but who are not in return receiving the opportunity and security promised by our arrangement of mutual rights and responsibilities. The elderly and essential workers, for instance, have been left exposed to the pandemic. We have seen disparate impacts on communities of color, because underlying foundations of health have not been adequately established for low-income workers. When crisis hit, the society that promised to protect all did not in fact protect many of its members.

To repair our social contract, we need to understand the goals and responsibilities of public decision-makers and democratic citizens in a constitutional democracy in a time of crisis. We need to understand the vulnerabilities in our society that left us ill-equipped to fulfill those responsibilities. These are the subjects of chapter 1. We need to acknowledge what kind of public health strategy would have fulfilled those goals and responsibilities in response to this crisis, and we need to explore why we failed to adopt this strategy. These are the subjects of chapter 2. We need to learn how to use the machinery of our political institutions to deliver on those goals more effectively, if not now, in this crisis, then going forward. This is the subject of chapter 3. Once we take these steps, we will be able to sketch out the parameters of a transformed peace, a social contract that delivers pandemic resilience and, more generally, justice and health for our constitutional democracy on the foundation of a fair and flourishing economy. I offer that sketch in chapter 4.

Pandemic resilience requires public health infrastructure, of course, but also, and this will be my focus, a healthy social contract—good governance and bonds of solidarity and mutual commitment within the population, connected to love of country. Solidarity is the resource that enables people to make small sacrifices of liberty so as to avoid harm to others with whom they have a social bond. We convey our love of country through acts of solidarity to the other members of our polity. We have many reasons to want to benefit from a globally integrated economy and from the opportunities for human connection it brings. Yet we rightly wish to avoid being existentially vulnerable to its accompanying dangers. The goal is a framework for delivering a transformed peace, a postpandemic state in which, as a society, we would be less vulnerable to injury because we would be stronger as a society. We would have more civic strength by virtue of having a healthy social contract, supporting both good governance and solidarity.

1

Democracy in Crisis

The Problem to Be Solved

What goals of decision-making should guide a constitutional democracy in crisis? This chapter will answer that question but begins by sketching the nature of the emergency we confronted in January, February, and March 2020. The goal is to capture both how we saw the problem at the time of its emergence and how we *ought* to have seen the problem.

When the COVID-19 crisis hit, three kinds of problems quickly emerged: a health problem, an economic problem, and a political problem. The third, the political problem, is the focus of this book. In order to come to grips with it, though, it will be necessary to say something briefly about the two problems with which it interacts, the health and the economic problems. The job facing our political institutions in January 2020 was to solve those intersecting challenges. As I finished this book in March 2021, there were more than five hundred thousand Americans dead, we had the highest death toll in the world, the majority of the nation's schools were still functioning remotely, and severe economic impacts were and still are visible in dramatic increases in food insecurity (GAO 2020), women who have dropped out of the workforce (Cohen 2020), and a rising tide of evictions (Badger 2020). Many would agree that the United States failed to meet the moment by mounting either a successful response to COVID-19 or achieving pandemic resilience.

To know how and why our institutions failed, we need to understand the task that lay before them at the start of 2020. A first issue here is whether constitutional democracies have what it takes to deliver a solution to health and economic problems of the kind presented by a rapidly moving pandemic. By now we know the answer is yes. New Zealand, Australia, Taiwan, Germany, and South Korea all handled the crisis reasonably well, minimizing death and negative economic impacts and preserving liberties. The problem faced in the United States will turn out not to reflect weaknesses of constitutional democracy per se but weaknesses in the United States specifically.

In what follows, I will sketch the key intellectual mistakes we made in our approach to COVID-19. These were (1) the assumption of a trade-off between the protection of health and the protection of the economy and (2) a failure to learn from others. I will argue that we ought instead to have framed our decision-making with the goal of maximizing alignment among the goals of securing lives, livelihoods, and liberties. Constitutional democracies, I will argue, require a distinctive kind of decision-making and judgment, even in a crisis. It is the goal of this chapter to make that special feature of constitutional democracy visible.

Existential Threat, Not Utilitarian Costs and Benefits

The general public first became aware of COVID-19's arrival in the United States with cases in Washington State in February. (We now know that there were earlier cases on the West Coast as early as December 2019; Basavaraju 2020.) Given the scale of devastation in Italy in particular, it was clear from mid-February onward that there was potential for significant numbers of deaths in the United States—initial projections estimated as many as two million people if the disease were to proceed unchecked through the population. Modeling from multiple epidemiological groups pointed in this direction.[1]

It also soon became clear that countries with strong national health systems—such as Germany—were not only achieving a lower caseload but also keeping mortality lower. As we discovered more about the high infection and fatality rate in poorer and minority communities in the United States, it began to look as if a realistic estimate of our potential toll might actually be on the order of three million dead. We were, in short, facing loss of life on a scale greater than that of many wars the country has fought. In terms of relative population, the loss of life had the potential to reach half the tally for the Civil War. Moreover, it was clear that the loss was going to rip through our population in ways that tracked quite profound and historically long-standing health and economic inequities. Stark disparities along racial and ethnic lines ensured that the pandemic would play out as a tale of two different countries.

The speed of the virus's spread, combined with its degree of fatality, introduced the possibility that our health infrastructure would be overwhelmed. We would simply not have sufficient medical resources to meet exponentially accelerating need, let alone to continue medical care for all of the other issues that afflict our population on an annual basis. This was an existential threat. Health care and public health institutions

---

1. Estimates for deaths in 2020 ranged from 240,000 from the Institute for Health Metrics and Evaluation to 2.2 million from Imperial College (Ferguson et al. 2020), with the latter number projecting a death toll in the event that no measures at all were taken to impede the progress of the disease.

are among the core pillars of any functioning society. If they cease to function, they will bring with them a cascade of other problems of legitimacy. A society that cannot keep its hospitals functioning will quickly see a collapse in perceived legitimacy of political leadership and possibly of political institutions also.[2] This was the health problem we faced in late February and early March.

At the time the crisis hit, our public health professionals had one tool in the toolbox for staving off this existential challenge: collective stay-at-home orders. And so we entered into a national lockdown in the middle of March.

Yet this in turn provoked a second existential threat. Collective stay-at-home orders were a necessary response to the immediate crisis because we had uncertain knowledge about the overall shape of the disease. Yet the weapon that could kill rapidly traveling viruses also kills economies. Both viruses and economies depend on active, frequent social interactions. The primary tool in the public health toolbox worked well, it turned out, only against localized epidemics. Localized stay-at-home orders take one bit of the economy off-line at a time, leaving the rest in operation to sustain even the portion temporarily closed. But global stay-at-home orders? They led to the most severe economic collapse since the Great Depression. In the United States, the collective national quarantine of March and April cost $350 billion a month. Gross domestic product (GDP) decreased 32 percent in the second quarter of the year, and that drop was accompanied by steep job losses that will have long-term consequences for those who suddenly fell into unemployment (Bureau of Economic Analysis 2020).

2. For some examples, see McDowall and Basma 2017; Schaart, Bayer, and Jennings 2019; WHO 2009. See also Clinton administration health reform efforts, which led to the 1994 Republican Contract with America.

Applied simultaneously across the globe, collective stay-at-home orders were just as existentially threatening as the disease itself. The discipline of public health was not ready for a truly globalized, highly infectious, highly dangerous pathogen. Its emergence cried out for innovation and invention, and for the discovery of new public health tools compatible with a functioning economy.

Yet this is not what we got. Instead, our national political discourse settled into a reflexive discussion about whether to choose health or the economy, in short "lives" or "livelihoods." Yet that talk of trade-off was badly misconceived. We did not work from a stable institutional and decision-making environment in which we could balance risks of different kinds and make fine-grained calculations of the trade-offs. To the contrary, the threat to our basic institutions—specifically, our public health institutions—but also to the legitimacy of our institutions more generally—was severe enough to force the question of how to secure the foundations of a functioning society. The necessary frame for decision-making was not the utilitarian cost-benefit calculations of an accountant with a green eyeshade but the kind of deliberation familiar in wartime. The question was not how to trade off lives and livelihoods but how to secure the foundations of our society by securing lives and livelihoods simultaneously (Allen, Stanczyk, et al. 2020).

Of course, we were not actually fighting a war. Nonetheless, the relevant orientation for moral decision-making was quite consistent with a wartime context and just war theory. In wartime, the goal is to defend lives and livelihoods simultaneously. A society can succeed in the face of the existential threat of wartime only if it has a functioning economy. Even more importantly, in wartime, the job is *to mobilize the economy in order to fight the war* effectively and thus secure lives. Protecting life requires protecting the economy. The two goals are integrated and aligned. The question is not one of trade-offs but of how to find pathways to that integration and alignment. When the COVID-19 crisis hit, we needed modes of analysis that began by recognizing the integration and alignment of our goals and that sought the tactics necessary to deliver on that alignment. In short, we needed a tool for fighting the virus that would not also shut down the economy, and we needed to mobilize the economy to deliver that tool.

That tool was not hard to discover. Asian nations were already using it: a massive ramp-up of diagnostic testing for the disease coupled with massively scaled-up contact tracing. Those contact-tracing teams would not only rapidly follow up on all cases and ensure that those who were exposed to the disease were isolated, they would also make sure the quarantined were provided supports to isolate for a sufficient time to block the onward transmission of the virus. We might have had innovation and invention for our public health infrastructure, if only we had been willing to look to models outside our own borders.

Two intellectual problems, then, characterized our early response. First, we defaulted to utilitarian trade-off modes of analysis rather than recognizing the existential threat and asking the more fundamental question of how to secure the stability of our institutions by aligning our efforts to protect lives and livelihoods. Second, we remained resolutely unwilling to follow the examples set by those outside our own borders. In mid-April, my research network called the head of the German disease control agency to ask about the public health infrastructure they were building, and we learned from him that it was uncommon to get a call from Americans.

Had our country been willing to learn from others and to bring the spirit of wartime deliberations to our work in early March, we might have pursued a very rapid recomposition of the economy to deliver the tools of testing and contact tracing at massive scale. That would have permitted us to fight the disease with methods like those used in Asian nations, for example, South Korea. No laws of physics had to be broken to accomplish this. This has led many to suggest that the roots of our failure to invest rapidly in our public health infrastructure were political and cultural.

In those early days of crisis, with a solution visible plain as day in other countries, many blamed the United States' flailing efforts on our federal system and strong culture of individual rights. They argued that a decentralized system of government that devolves significant power to fifty states is no match for a fast-acting virus (Horgan 2020). Those who espoused this view often pointed to China's prompt response to the outbreak as a model for decision-making in a crisis, arguing that only a centralized authoritarian state can act quickly and ruthlessly enough to squelch the virus, even if trampling over civil liberties to do so. But this overlooks that both Australia and Germany, with federal systems, succeeded in responding to the virus. Neither democracy nor federalism was the problem. Indeed, federalism is an asset and could have been of great value to us if we had taken more advantage of its resources. Similarly, Germany and Taiwan have some of the most privacy-protective rights regimes in the world. Vigorous defense of liberties hindered the response in neither country.

Yet it is true that the path to success involved breaking laws— not of physics but of politics. The work that had to be done in the United States—and in Germany and Australia—was different in kind than the work China needed to do. The challenge facing us was distinctive to constitutional democracies. A successful response to existential threats requires not merely survival but survival as the kind of society we are. The United States needed to rise to the existential threats it faced not as a generic society but as the specific kind of society it is, namely a constitutional democracy. This country, like Australia and Germany, needed to secure not just life and livelihood but also liberty, all simultaneously. Yes, we needed to shake loose the hold of technocratic cost-benefit analyses, and we also needed to slip from the grip of our own parochialism. We also needed, however, to achieve a deeper understanding of the specificities of the problem that faced us as a constitutional democracy. We needed a response to those aspects specifically.

Distinctive demands are made on constitutional democracies by a crisis. I turn to that topic now. In 2020, to understand and act on those demands would have required breaking the laws of politics.

Crisis and Political Legitimacy

What were the stakes of this crisis for constitutional democracy in general and for our democracy in particular? All decent regimes face the challenge of responding to existential threats by restoring security and well-being for their populace. One of the most ancient distinctions among regime types is simply that between well-ordered and outlaw regimes. The former pursue basic security for their populace. The latter don't. The distinction goes back to Plato and Aristotle.

Plato and Aristotle argued that the first criterion for judging how well a given regime performed was simply whether the rulers were acting in the interest of the ruled or in their own inter-

TABLE 1. Diversity of the world's regime types: First distinction

	Regime category	Basic material security
Well-ordered regimes	Democracies and decent authoritarian regimes	Y
Outlaw regimes	Nondecent, rights-violating regimes	N

est. In every good regime—regardless of whether ruled by one, few, or many—rulers rule for the sake of the people being ruled and therefore deliver basic well-being to the population. This is the first requirement for political legitimacy of any kind. In the United States, this requirement is articulated in the Declaration of Independence, when that text defines the first principle of our institutions as being that we build them in order to "effect [our] safety and happiness," that is, our *collective* safety and happiness.[3] The phrase, which comes at the end of the long second sentence about self-evident truths, is an eighteenth-century rendering of Cicero's argument that "the health of the people is the supreme law" (*salus populi suprema lex esto*). Both the phrase "safety and happiness" in the Declaration and the phrase "general welfare" in the preamble to the US Constitution are eighteenth-century renderings of this Roman idea. The Declaration does not treat our individual pursuit of happiness as the point of our political institutions. Instead it argues that people build their political institutions to achieve their shared safety and happiness, one element of which consists of providing a context in which people can autonomously pursue the life courses they choose ("the pursuit of happiness"). From antiquity through the founding of the United States, political theorists have consistently argued that all political legitimacy flows from the ability of political institutions to deliver the

---

3. "We hold these truths to be self-evident: That all men are created equal; that they are endowed by their Creator with certain unalienable rights; that among these are life, liberty, and the pursuit of happiness; that, to secure these rights, governments are instituted among men, deriving their just powers from the consent of the governed; that whenever any form of government becomes destructive of these ends, it is the right of the people to alter or to abolish it, and to institute new government, laying its foundation on such principles, and organizing its powers in such form, as to them shall seem most likely to effect their safety and happiness."

health and well-being of the people as a collective body. Success at providing material security is a necessary element of legitimacy for any regime type.

The COVID-19 crisis, then, threatened all political regimes on earth with legitimacy failure should it be the case that they could not master the disease and deliver material security to their populations. To make matters worse for us, in the United States this threat to legitimacy arrived at a time when our political institutions were already facing a legitimacy crisis. When the pandemic hit, we did not have broad consensus that our institutions were delivering the basic material security that we collectively need. That issue comes to the fore most powerfully and sharply in the opinions of young people. Whereas for the generation born before World War II, roughly 70 percent consider it essential to live in a democracy, for millennials, only about 30 percent consider it so (Foa and Mounk 2016). Or if they're asked whether a democratic system is a good or bad way to run a country, 25 percent of young people will say it's a bad or very bad way to run a country.

Both climate change and economic inequality are commonly invoked by young voters to explain their disaffection with and alienation from our political institutions. With regard to both issues, young people express the view that older generations have abandoned them to an existentially unsustainable existence. Even before the COVID-19 crisis hit, we had lost the allegiance of rising generations to our system of governance. The question, then, of whether this country could respond reasonably and effectively to the COVID-19 crisis and satisfactorily deliver a basic sense of material safety and security went right to the heart of what was already a legitimacy crisis.

Yet the achievement of material security is only the beginning of the story of democratic legitimacy. Constitutional democracies also have their own additional conditions for achieving and maintaining legitimacy. I turn to those now.

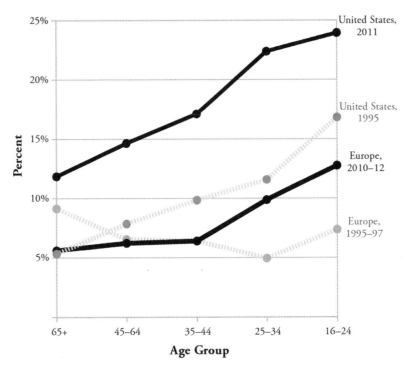

FIGURE 1. Percentage of respondents who said having a democratic political system is a "bad" or "very bad" way to run the country, by age group and location

SOURCE: Foa and Mounk 2016

The premise underlying democracy is that human flourishing extends beyond basic material security. Such security is necessary but not sufficient. Human beings, in the common account of the value of democracy, are creatures who need to chart their own courses in life. They thrive on autonomy, the opportunity for self-creation and self-governance. That autonomy is made real in our political institutions via the protection of both negative and positive liberties. Negative liberties are those rights of free speech, rights of association, rights of freedom of religion and so forth, that permit us each to chart our own course toward happiness, based on our own definitions of the good. Positive liberties and rights are those opportunities that we have to participate in our political institutions as decision-makers, as voters, as elected officials, as people who contribute to the deliberations of our public bodies. Through our positive liberties, we have the chance to shape our collective world together. A core insight of democratic theory is that the autonomy that delivers human flourishing also requires a second kind of shared autonomy through political institutions in order for autonomy to have its fullest form. To focus on material security alone leads to only a partial flourishing; a fuller flourishing requires also the protection and exercise of negative and positive liberties. Beyond that, too, full flourishing requires protection of social rights that interact with basic material security to make sure that we have that foundation of economic opportunity and possibility that permits us to make use of our negative and positive liberties.

This account of flourishing, which sees human well-being as extending beyond the material, has led to further categorizations of regime types beyond the basic distinction between well-ordered and outlaw regimes. Over the course of the twentieth century, regimes have been categorized depending on whether they focused only on material security, or also on negative liberties, positive liberties, and social rights.

China, for example, would be a society where the political institutions and authorities are committed to the material well-being of good parts of their population (though not to the well-being of minorities such as the Uighurs). The Chinese government is also committed to a certain provision of social rights—health rights, for example—but not to negative liberties or positive rights. Insofar as the leaders are governing in the interest of achieving material security, China falls into the category of well-ordered regimes, but not into the category of constitutional democracies, which must also protect negative and positive rights and liberties.

TABLE 2. Diversity of the world's regime types: Twentieth-century frame

	Regime category	Basic material security	Negative liberties/ rights	Positive liberties/ rights	Social rights
Well-ordered regimes	Egalitarian participatory democracy	Y	Y	Y	Y
	Constitutional democracy	Y	Y	Y	Y
	Rights-protecting autocratic regimes	Y	Y	N	Y
	Material well-being–protecting authoritarian/ autocratic regimes	Y	N	N	Y
Outlaw regimes	Nondecent, rights-violating regimes	N	N	N	N

Yet even these categorizations are insufficient to have a full picture of the legitimacy challenge facing the United States before COVID-19 hit. The twenty-first century has given us a further requirement for legitimacy in constitutional democracies. In addition to protecting negative and positive liberties, a healthy constitutional democracy must also secure social equality and nondiscrimination in order that positive and negative rights and liberties, as well as social rights, are equally well secured for all members of the polity.

Long-standing patterns of discrimination undermine the provision of negative liberties, positive liberties, and social rights, as we have at long last come to understand. Consequently, achieving the core goals of a constitutional democracy also requires focusing on issues of social equality and nondiscrimination. As health inequities became visible in this coronavirus

TABLE 3. Diversity of the world's regime types: Twenty-first-century frame

	Regime category	Basic material security	Negative liberties/ rights	Positive liberties/ rights	Social rights	Social equality/ nondiscrimination
Well-ordered regimes	Egalitarian participatory democracy	Y	Y	Y	Y	Y
	Constitutional democracy	Y	Y	Y	Y	?
	Rights-protecting autocratic regimes	Y	Y	N	Y	?
	Material well-being–protecting authoritarian/ autocratic regimes	Y	N	N	Y	?
Outlaw regimes	Nondecent, Rights-violating regimes	N	N	N	N	N

pandemic, they made abundantly clear how tenuous was the legitimacy of our political institutions.

In the twenty-first century, as we seek to renew our understanding of the value of democracy and to set our aspirations on a higher target for its realization, inequities of the kind that have been exposed through the pandemic reveal a social contract that is fundamentally compromised. Securing material well-being, securing *salus populi*, the happiness and safety of the people, requires securing that for everyone. And securing that for all requires that we constantly revisit our processes, our organizations, our forms of distribution, to see that we have achieved them through equality and nondiscrimination. A constitutional democracy must navigate through crisis not merely by responding to the threat to security but also by doing so in such a way that it can survive as the kind of society it seeks to be: one that pursues and protects negative liberties, positive liberties, social rights, and social equality. These are the high standards to which a democracy must remain faithful even when it faces a crisis.

The higher bar constitutional democracies set for their decision-making, including in times of crisis, leads to distinctive requirements of governance. Precisely because a constitutional democracy faces a harder set of tasks, it needs a distinctive approach to governance to deliver on those tasks.

Four specific responsibilities of governance come to the fore when we focus on all of the different aspects of legitimacy that are not only necessary but also, when taken together, sufficient to support a constitutional democracy. These responsibilities are (1) integrative policy-making and judgment; (2) education of the public; (3) attention to a healthy social contract via protection of negative and positive liberties; and (4) attention to a healthy social contract via protection of social rights, social equality, and nondiscrimination.

As we have seen, legitimacy in a constitutional democracy depends on success at securing material well-being, protecting negative liberties, protecting positive liberties, protecting social rights, and securing social equality. Decisions have to be integrated across all of these dimensions. This requires partnerships among experts in each area. There is a need for expertise on the specific issues of material security in play. In the case of the pandemic, we needed experts on health and economics to help shape our policy conversation. But they have to be fully integrated with and collaborating with experts in law, focused on civil liberties; experts working on questions of equity and social policy; experts working on questions of community health and how questions of health equity factor into the overall shape of a policy. In that regard, precisely because constitutional democracies need to work out any decision across a number of dimensions, they need leaders who are like symphony conductors—able to activate the different instruments needed for judgment across many dimensions simultaneously, and to weave those different instruments together into an integrated whole.

Such leaders also need to guide education of the public. The existence of our positive liberties, the fact that we, the people, ultimately are the rulers in this democracy, means that public decisions require our support and our understanding. The commitment of a democracy to positive liberties brings with it a commitment to transparency in communication. During a time of fast-moving crisis, this amounts to a commitment to clear and consistent public education. In order for citizens of a democracy to see and understand the crisis, the integrative process of diagnosing the crisis's components and of finding solution pathways needs to be shared with the public in ways that make the choices before us visible. We need public officials who can explain the pursuit of alignment along all the dimensions of our aspirations and explain how integration will be achieved.

This celebration of public education by politicians may raise certain familiar worries. For instance, how is public education, in this context, different from public relations, or even propaganda? Once experts, including expert policy-makers, have taken an action, don't they develop an interest in defending themselves, which may or may not be consistent with the public's interest?

In fact, the work of public education should *precede* the taking of the decision. Education isn't something that becomes necessary simply when officials are ready to announce a decision. Instead, public officials should educate the public throughout the process of deliberation. The public should have the opportunity to learn exactly what question decision-makers seek to answer and how they will go about it. Then, as public officials close in on an answer, they should educate the public on the developments in their thinking, so that when they announce the decision, they do so on the basis of a whole sequence of prior educative moments.

The distinction between education and propaganda is maintained by a commitment of elected officials to truthfulness. We have a big debate in our country about facts, and often people lament that we don't all seem to be operating with the same set of facts. That's not quite the right diagnosis of our problem. The question of which evidence is salient to a decision will depend on what question you're trying to ask and answer; so part of the process of debate will inevitably involve a contest over which facts are the most important ones. When people try to nail down a single set of agreed-upon facts, as if that will bring an end to problematic debate, they often find the project immensely elusive. Antipropaganda efforts in the lead-up to World War II faced this problem (Allen and Pottle 2018). What matters is not that we stabilize a set of facts as the ones that we'll all agree to focus on but that we stabilize a widespread commitment to truthfulness. This commitment is needed to undergird any understanding of evidence and argumentation. A commitment to truthfulness is, at the end of the day, what distinguishes education from propaganda.

What institutions do we have that can foster a commitment to truthfulness, especially in this moment? There is, after all, much distrust in the media and in universities. This is a very hard problem, and the question of how to reverse the erosion of an ethic of truthfulness is not straightforward. That said, there are some wonderful innovators showing the way. In Lexington, Kentucky, an organization called CivicLex has invented what I have taken to calling "civic media" to contrast it with "social media." If social media is like permanent middle school with incessant bullying and trolling, civic media is what we can grow into. At CivicLex, they've taken on themselves the job of building a fresh architecture of explanatory and investigative journalism at the local level and also of providing meeting places where public officials and citizens can come together, in a ratio of never more than one official to every seven citizens. They have brought high journalistic standards to this work and are educating their community, Lexington, about those standards, and engaging people across the community in the work of rebuilding shareable, usable civic knowledge. The seven-to-one ratio for the in-person gatherings means that people have to focus on the quality of the relationships they have with one another. People are processing information in relational contexts that demand interpersonal responsibility. There is a hunger in our society for an alternative to the media universe in which we all live. Civic-Lex is giving people in Lexington, Kentucky, information that they need, in a social context that permits establishing sound norms. The question is how we can take good experiments like this, strengthen them, and spread them so that collectively we can rebuild an understanding of the work of building up solid usable knowledge, and a commitment to truthfulness.

The third important responsibility of democratic governance is attention to a healthy social contract via protection of negative and positive liberties. Our commitment to positive and negative liberties means that in responding to this crisis, some of the tools in use in other societies are off limits. For instance, both China and South Korea have used intense surveillance tools to track and quarantine people in order to control the disease. South Korea has centralized a variety of health and credit card data in order to track COVID-19 cases and their possible transmission. The level of data surveillance being conducted in these countries violates fundamental commitments to privacy that serve to protect autonomy in constitutional democracies.

Similarly, China has routinely quarantined vast swaths of the population to a much greater extent than we have here in the United States. It has enforced these quarantines with tools that are incompatible with the protection of civil liberties, including location data, facial recognition technology, and QR codes that hang over the entrance to residential complexes, used to support tracking of people's movements (Yang et al. 2020).

While state public health emergency powers in the United States include the authority to issue quarantine orders that are legally enforceable, public health authorities have historically sought to avoid broad imposition of sanction-bearing mandates in order to keep the impact on civil liberties to a minimum. Given reluctance to rely on tools that conflict with civil liberties, officials in constitutional democracies must instead rely on another tool: voluntaristic participation resting on solidarity, a commitment of the citizenry to undertake burdens on one another's behalf. The fact that democracies have a higher bar for building and sustaining legitimacy means that, when they succeed, they also have resources of solidarity in the population to tap, so that supportive volunteerism can be activated on behalf of the public good. But as political scientists will point out, the resources of solidarity depend on a functioning and healthy social contract (Cammett and Lieberman 2020). The question of how a democracy meets a crisis when it needs to use stringent measures— and how well it succeeds at that—will closely interact with the health of the social contract: whether or not the basic relations among the citizenry, the existing forms of mutual commitment themselves, can shore up the kind of solidarity it takes to do hard things together in a time of crisis.

The fourth and final feature of legitimate democratic governance is attention to a healthy social contract via protection of social rights, social equality, and nondiscrimination. This responsibility highlights the importance of continuously tending to the health of the social contract itself—the health of relations among the citizenry and the provision of foundations for flourishing equally for all. When either of those two dimensions of the social contact weakens, the capacity of the society to respond to moments of crisis will also weaken. In this crisis, we've all seen many ways our social contract is weaker than we might have thought. As we discover these weaknesses, we have to recognize that they also identify places where our resources, our supplies of solidarity and supportive volunteerism, are not as full and rich as we would ideally like them to be.

What do these four responsibilities add up to? In order to navigate through a crisis, constitutional democracies need the capacity to identify and organize around a common purpose. The four elements of governance discussed here are the processes needed to build that common purpose.

Not only in crises but also generally, democratic governance fundamentally is about creating a sense of common purpose. By "sense of common purpose," I mean an affective connection to a common enterprise, but I also intend to convey a clear understanding of the content of a shared goal. Many may think that the prospect of a "common purpose," particularly in a mass democracy of more than three hundred million people, is simply the silly romantic notion of a sentimental democrat. But a common purpose is not an airy-fairy thing. It's a practical tool that permits people to achieve something together (Finnemore and Jurkovich 2020). A common purpose is a map marked with a destination, a guide that permits coordination and collaborative navigation. It's probably the most powerful tool in the democratic tool kit, particularly in a crisis, because it is common purpose that can yield solidarity and that enables people to do hard things voluntarily rather than through authoritarian compulsion.

How do the four aspects of governance relate to a common purpose?

Integrative judgment supports the discovery of what it is we should do. It gives content to the purpose that should set our strategic direction. Rather than having a conversation where one expert argues for the tool which suits that expertise best and another for a tool that belongs to another domain of expertise, we have to look for the questions that rise above the domains of expertise. The questions we faced in March with the coronavirus were not purely health questions. They were not purely economic questions. They were rather questions of how we could secure the foundations of a healthy society, a society that protects health and mobilizes the economy to do that. That formulation of an integrative question is a necessary thing for the development of a common purpose. It's the question that is used to lay out a track to a shared destination. The job of identifying policy solutions, then, is about figuring out what that common-purpose policy is, the integrative response that identifies needs across domains and figures out how to align and combine them.

Public education supports common purpose by turning that strategic purpose into something shared or common. The public is invited into that process of diagnosis, that effort to understand the circumstances in which we find ourselves and to see how the different domains of expertise come together to inform our core decisions. As a solutions pathway emerges, the point of public education is to ensure that people can see together that the pathway we're choosing is one inspired by a common purpose, the need to pursue and achieve our shared aspirations as a society as a whole, not the aspirations for public health, not the aspirations for economics, not the aspirations for Texas, the aspirations for New York, but rather a shared vision of what it means to set our world to rights together.

Then a common purpose is useful to us because it should deliver on a social contract, not only by achieving material security but also by securing positive and negative liberties and rights, social rights, and social equality. Ultimately if we are able to identify a common purpose, we will know it precisely because it offers a solution pathway that lays out a path to material security while also protecting liberties and rights, social rights, and social equality. The only sound measure, I think, of democratic decision-making in a time of crisis is whether it achieves all those things simultaneously.

"Common purpose" is the name for that kind of integration of thinking. It is also the name for the process of public education that we need as a society to be able to pull together, tapping into the resources of solidarity, to do the hard things that will protect lives, livelihoods, and liberties simultaneously.

Our Vulnerabilities

With these aspects of democratic governance now clearly before us, we can see our own vulnerabilities more sharply. I've alluded to some of them already, and none will surprise you. Our vulnerabilities are perhaps what pressed themselves upon us most powerfully in 2020.

The vulnerabilities revealed by the pandemic did not really have to do with whether we were ready for a crisis of this specific kind, a SARS-like experience of the coronavirus, as opposed to influenza or something of that sort. That is, the story of our vulnerabilities is not about whether we were insufficiently prepared for this disease in particular. *The question is whether our constitutional democracy was prepared for any crisis of any kind whatsoever*. Were our resources of democratic resilience already tapped out when this crisis hit?

We faced serious challenges and, in relation to all four of the necessary elements of democratic governance laid out above, we came up wanting. It's worth looking at the specifics of those challenges with regard to the need to achieve integrative pol-

icy, public education, and a healthy social contract—along the
dimensions of both rights protection and social equality.

Let's start with the need for integrative policy work. Since
February, we've had a public argument about whether we should
listen to public health experts or economists. This is the wrong
way to go about the question. Public health experts have only
part of the answer. They know how to fight diseases. Similarly,
economists have only a separate part of the answer. They know
how to keep liquidity flowing or how to stimulate a sinking
economy. But public health experts in February had no reason
or training to ask questions about political economy such as
"Can this economy in a compressed time period deliver a testing infrastructure such as this country has never seen before?"
With no context for asking that question, public health experts
had no reason to imagine tools of disease response that would
depend on that kind of economic capacity.

Similarly, economists had no reason or training to ask questions such as "Is there a tool for disease control other than
collective stay-at-home orders that might be less damaging to
the economy?" Economists don't ask questions about how to
solve health problems. Public health experts don't ask questions about how to transform the structure of supply chains.
There was a pressing need to integrate the policy space, to take
in advice from experts in each area, and then to make integrative judgments. Our failure to achieve this reveals our need to
shake off the shackles of deference to technocracy. Our leaders
should have led us in asking the right questions, and then making judgment calls, taking into account the best advice experts
could give but recognizing that that's all that experts do: give
advice. It's the job of elected leaders to see the integrative problem and find the integrative solution.

What about public education? How well have the American people been led through a transparent, well-structured

decision-making process? How clearly have our actual choices
been presented to us? Here our record is abysmal, and this was
thanks largely to the conduct of then President Trump. The
presidency is the single most powerful teaching platform in the
country. President Donald Trump, the person with the greatest power to educate the public and motivate the whole country
behind a common purpose, not only declined to use that power,
but even spewed misinformation into the public conversation
in steady streams. This was a personal failing, but it was not
just that. It was also the single greatest institutional obstacle to
successful response. To implement a crisis plan, leaders need
to activate the machinery of government and do the nuts-and-
bolts work of setting policies and directing resources. But the
machinery of government is greased by the smoothing oil of
public acceptance. And acceptance is won by respecting the
public's need to understand and by respecting the intelligence
of the public.

One lesson of the 2020 pandemic is that no amount of civil
society effort from nongovernmental organizations to provide
clear, calm, reasoned information, even if exceptionally well
and broadly coordinated, can counterbalance chaotic, inco-
herent, constantly changing communication from the White
House. Crisis communication from the White House should be
conducted, at a minimum, to the same standard as we expect
every classroom educator to meet: acknowledge the emotional
moment, clearly and crisply frame the analytical work to be
done, articulate the overarching moral concerns at stake in the
moment, and make a case to the American people for the role
each can play in resolving the crisis. Ensure steadiness of purpose and of inquiry throughout the course of the crisis.

At one level, the choice to be presented to the American
people should have been incredibly simple. The tool we needed
to control the disease was a combination of universal precau-

tions like mask-wearing and testing at scale. This two-pronged response had public health validity. It had economic viability. It could have kept schools open.

But even with clarity about these tools, there would have been further choices and decisions requiring clear communication to the American people. How much testing should a community have? The answer to that depended on what goals any given community might choose for its testing program. The choice of goals is where the work of integrating perspectives happens. Three goals circulated through policy discussions without ever explicitly being named. Some policy proposals were built around the goal of using testing mainly for therapeutic purposes to help treat those who were sick. Some were built around the goal of using testing for purposes of contact tracing to help suppress COVID-19 and remove it from the community but to do so as one tool among many others, for example, stay-at-home orders. Some policies were built around the goal of using testing and contact tracing as a tool of disease suppression powerful enough itself to eliminate the disease and keep second waves at bay. The CDC guidance on testing blended all three of these purposes together and was never articulated in a fashion that made the need for a strategic choice of objective clear.

Each of these purposes—a therapeutic purpose; a minimal testing and contact-tracing purpose; and a maximal testing and contact-tracing purpose—required a different level of testing and would have made different demands on the testing supply chain. Effective activation of the supply chain would have required a clear decision about which strategy to pursue. Elected officials needed to make a judgment call and to explain it to the American people. They needed to answer the question of which approach to testing we should pursue. This never occurred throughout 2020. In the absence of clear strategic objectives, we failed throughout the whole course of 2020 to complete the activation of our testing supply chain. During Thanksgiving week, eleven months into the pandemic, we saw a nationwide surge of the disease and people waiting days to get a COVID-19 test (Moore 2020). Not only did Americans go without what they needed, the American people were left in confusion about the role and place of testing, contact tracing, and supported isolation in mastering the challenge of COVID-19. The failure to establish a clear strategic objective, and the resulting failure of public education, were the most profound shortcomings of our COVID-19 response.

With regard to the third aspect of governance, the question of whether our social contract is healthy enough for us to tap into resources of solidarity, there, too, the challenges we faced are clear. We faced both polarization and racial disparities. The story is familiar. Figure 2 shows some basic data about changing political viewpoints in our country and how Republicans and Democrats have moved farther apart over time.

The chart in figure 2 ends in 2017, and as we all know the situation has grown only more severe since then, resulting in 2020 in another election with a populace almost evenly split between two presidential candidates of strikingly different types.

With regard to health inequities, figures 3 and 4 provide some information on the disparate impacts of COVID-19 on different communities in this country. The chart shown in figure 3 captures data from New York City with the number of deaths per hundred thousand people as of April 22, 2020. The lower panel is adjusted by age, and therefore it takes into account the fact that the population of the United States in older generations includes a higher percentage of white people. That is, insofar as COVID-19 has a much more significant impact on people over seventy, when adjusted for the generational component of COVID-19 impacts, the bottom graph gives a sense of how disparate impacts are playing out specifically by race.

Growing gaps between Republicans and Democrats across domains

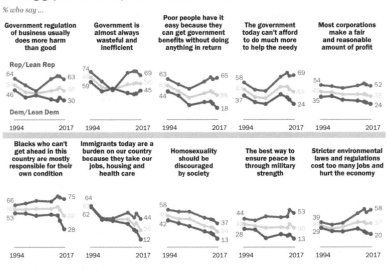

FIGURE 2. Polarization

SOURCE: Pew Research Center 2017; survey conducted June 8–18 and June 27–July 9, 2017

The chart shown in figure 4 captures data from around the country. The disparate impacts by race are very closely connected to socioeconomic disparities. The racial disparities are less severe where socioeconomic disparities are not as great. But where socioeconomic disparities are great, we see more severe disparities in the impact of COVID-19 on African American communities than on other communities. Of course, the brutal police killing of George Floyd and the summer protests that followed further highlighted how badly rent our social fabric is with regard to the demands of racial justice.

When we see data of this kind—on polarization, on health inequity, on police violence in relation to communities of color—these are red alerts that our social contract is failing to nourish solidarity, failing to secure well-being for all, and

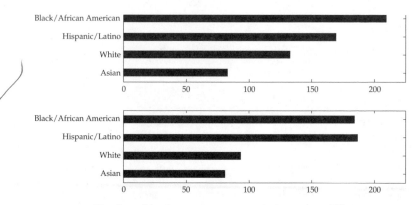

FIGURE 3. Number of deaths per 100,000 population among different ethnic groups as of April 22, 2020, in New York City: *top*, unadjusted data; *bottom*, adjusted by age

SOURCE: Figure from Sethi et al. 2020; data from New York City Department of Health and Mental Hygiene

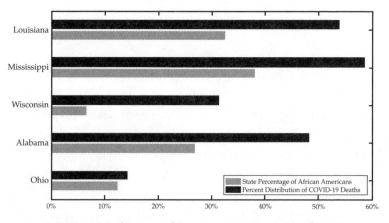

FIGURE 4. Disparities between African American proportion of COVID-19 deaths and African American proportion of population in states with lowest African American median income as of May 2020

SOURCE: Figure from Sethi et al. 2020; data from New York City Department of Health and Mental Hygiene

failing to secure the basic foundation for the sets of liberties needed for full human flourishing. When we see such red alerts about the quality and health of our social contract, we should recognize that achieving solidarity at a moment of crisis will be challenging. These data reflect civic weakness instead of the civic strength that any constitutional democracy needs if it is going to find sources of resilience in the face of a crisis.

In a crisis, a constitutional democracy will succeed to the degree that its leaders can cultivate common purpose. But if a constitutional democracy meets a moment of crisis at a time when there are substantial ruptures in the social contract, then finding common purpose requires not only an integrative policy solution to the existential threat at hand but also ways to reweave the social contract in a healthy form. To defeat the virus, we actually need to rebuild our social contract so that we have the resources of solidarity necessary to master the moment. This means that the challenge of beating down the impacts of COVID-19 is not a short-term one. We won't be through this crisis until we have been able to build up new stores of resilience by reweaving our social contract and achieving enough civic strength to sustain the whole population.

We have seen that the initial challenge to a constitutional democracy from COVID-19 was not merely the need for effective policy to control the disease and keep the economy open. The necessary policy framework was already in existence in other countries. The real challenge—and the one at which we failed in the United States—was for integrated judgment explained with sound, consistent public education. No laws of physics had to be broken to achieve a sound policy pathway and the infrastructure of implementation. It was necessary, though, to break the laws of politics. The law of politics dictates that a constitutional democracy must have a strong social contract to support the governance resources it needs to meet a crisis. In

2020, the United States did not have that strong social contract, and so it lacked civic strength. Successful near-term response to the COVID-19 crisis would have required us to repair our social contract at a pace that only angels could have achieved. Mortals—moving in mortal temporal cadences—can repair frayed social bonds only with the speed at which trust can be grown. Politics has a physics as well, and that physics derives from the temporality of trust. Breaking the laws of politics proved impossible in the time available to us in 2020.

What should we do when the leaders of the government do not really believe in constitutional democracy? The good news is that in constitutional democracy, the origins of all power lie in the people. That continues to be true in the sense that popular opinion has a huge impact on what actually happens in Washington, DC. It's a very complicated dynamic between politics at the national level and how public opinion functions and operates. But it is within our power, as citizens, to build a conversation that we ourselves want and to drive that conversation into the spaces of decision-makers. Civil society matters. Civil society has power. The organizations of civil society can themselves take on the burden of rebuilding what we need.

A deeper healing of our social contract is needed if we are even to begin to invoke the idea of common purpose with any real seriousness. This pandemic has made plain that we are vulnerable because our democracy has grown weak with regard both to governance and the health of our social contract. A full response to COVID-19, then, and full achievement of pandemic resilience—or of crisis resilience more generally—will require that we learn again the core elements of successful democratic governance and find ways to heal our social contract of the damage done to it, by both inequity and polarization. Moreover, this will require work from all of us, not just our elected officials but all members of our society and our civil society organizations.

Chapters 2 and 3 lay out the path to pandemic resilience that we might have taken and further elaborate the forms of civic weakness that blocked our adoption of that pathway. Chapter 4 will lay out an agenda for healing our social contract, so that we can move forward to equip ourselves with the resources of civic strength that we needed when the crisis hit—and will no doubt need again in the future.

2

Pandemic Resilience

In Thucydides's *History of the Peloponnesian War*, the fine-grained, realist account of the late fifth-century BCE conflict in ancient Greece between democratic Athens and oligarchic Sparta, the general Pericles convinces rural Athenians to withdraw from their farms and to move inside the walls of the city. He hopes to ensure the Spartans will gain nothing from incursions into the Athenian countryside. Yet the tactic backfires when the density of people packed inside the city walls leads to the spread of a devastating plague, the death of a quarter of the population, and significant evisceration of Athens' fighting force. Pericles himself dies. This turn of affairs eventually leads to great political instability in Athens, and a second plague begins to emerge: dissension and polarization that leads the city ultimately to a civil war. The civil war in turn leads to defeat by Sparta.

The physical health of a population is a necessary foundation for a society's political and social health. The eighteenth-century political philosopher Jean-Jacques Rousseau argued that a single measure could show whether a society was flourishing: was its population growing?[1] While the pressures of

1. Jean-Jacques Rousseau, *Le Contrat Social*, bk. 3, chap. 9: "Des signes d'un bon Gouvernement": "Et quel est le signe le plus sûr qu'ils se conservent & prospèrent? C'est leur nombre & leur population."

massive global population growth give us a different view of that metric now, the basic point still stands. We know when a society is healthy just as we know when an apple orchard or herd of sheep is healthy: when the orchard or herd is productive and growing in number and when its individual members are able to live out full life spans in good health.

Of course, that apple orchard and sheep flock are healthy only when they are well nourished. So too with human populations. They must be nourished by a functional economy in order to be healthy at all. And typically health and economy are in a dynamic relationship to one another.

Pericles thought the Athenians could sacrifice part of their economy—their rural lands—without penalty in their fight against the Spartans, but his tactic disrupted the beneficial equilibrium supporting the economic and physical health of the city. The military leader did not recognize the need for practices to limit disease when, in wartime, the city's population density dramatically increased.

Similarly, in the case of COVID-19, the first response to the emergence of this highly infectious and therefore fast-moving pathogen was to use the most powerful tool in the public health toolkit: lockdowns shutting off social interaction. The principle of a lockdown to stop disease is similar to that proposed by Pericles: one sacrifices a portion of one's economy in order to preserve the functioning of the whole by protecting its health. Unfortunately, though, when a virus fully globalizes in a matter of months, and the lockdown closes most of the world's economy, the sacrifice itself is not contained. Instead the consequences are so thoroughgoing as to undermine the very capacity of the society to nourish and sustain itself.

In the context of a fully globalized world, where highly infectious diseases can travel as quickly to all corners of the globe as did COVID-19, we need to understand disease response differently than heretofore. We need an alternative approach that can defeat the disease by simultaneously limiting the number of cases and preserving functioning economies. That is, only such strategies to control the virus that also preserve economies are worth pursuing. In the case of the United States, the full national lockdown of March and April 2020 should have been used to establish the infrastructure we needed to fight COVID-19 while we waited for reinforcements in the form of an effective vaccine.

In order to protect lives, livelihoods, and liberties simultaneously, we should have built an infrastructure with five components: (1) a culture of adherence to universal precautions of mask-wearing and hand and bathroom hygiene supportive of infection control; (2) a supply chain and implementation infrastructure to support massively scaled-up diagnostic and screening testing, tracing, and supported isolation (TTSI) for those diagnosed as positive; (3) safely open schools; (4) a restoration of safety for in-person consumer services, like barbers, hair salons, and hotels, via screening testing; and (5) effective public communication.

In what follows, I will first review the features of the disease that created the parameters of possible responses. Then I will survey the initial policy responses that were mooted by experts. Next, I will lay out the five components of the pandemic response that we ought to have pursued; finally I will briefly address why we failed to adopt this strategy.

COVID-19: An Overview

By late December the United States passed a quarter of a million deaths, even before the end of 2020. This number was higher than the government's Coronavirus Task Force had projected as they tried to estimate the levels of mortality that would emerge given the strategies of response undertaken (Rucker and Wan 2020). In December 2020, we ranked fourteenth in deaths per capita (Belgium, Spain, Italy, and the UK were higher), and we had the largest absolute number of recorded COVID-19 deaths. In contrast to these other countries, Germany stood out as achieving Europe's most successful COVID-19 response (WHO 2020). Then vaccines arrived, a new chapter began, and the patterns shifted. But this book is about the prevaccine period.

For the original variants of COVID-19, the incubation period was up to two weeks. Median symptom onset came four to five days after exposure. This means that there was an extensive presymptomatic period, during which people were already infectious but potentially unaware of being so, leading to what epidemiologists call silent transmission. The number of asymptomatic and presymptomatic carriers who are able to infect others, because they don't know they are themselves infectious, has been estimated to be about 50 percent of cases throughout 2020 (CDC 2020b). That has been a significant part of the transmission story. Finally, COVID-19 fatality rates in 2020 were higher than for the flu, estimated at .05 percent in those over seventy, although only .00003 percent in those under nineteen. In 2020, the *observed* case fatality rate, a measure of the number of fatalities among confirmed cases, was 2 percent.

Herd immunity, the point at which there are no longer enough susceptible individuals in the population for the disease to continue spread, was, in 2020, typically understood to require 60 to 70 percent of the population to have been infected. To have a sense of the scale of impact required to achieve herd immunity in the absence of a vaccine, think back to the level of difficulty we saw in Italy in March 2020 and the overwhelmed state of their hospital system. By the end of March, only about 9 percent of the Italian population had been infected (Doi et al. 2020; Flaxman et al. 2020). At that time the UK was at about 2.7 percent infected. Even in really hard-hit areas, in other words, the level of immunity achieved prior to the arrival of vaccines was still far from the level needed for herd immunity.

In addition, science still has not yet resolved questions of whether antibodies provide durable immunity. We know they provide some immunity insofar as plasma with antibodies from people who have been exposed and recovered is a useful resource for treatment of those who are ill. We also know that the new vaccines that generate protective antibodies do prevent severe illness. What we don't know is how long that effect lasts. Is it short term? Is it longer term? Coronavirus immunity questions have been notoriously difficult as a matter of science.

In the COVID-19 pandemic, then, we faced (and continue to face) a highly infectious disease with an initially high but now declining fatality rate—and many open questions.

First Thoughts in February 2020

Two paradigms were immediately mooted as possible responses when the pandemic hit the United States. One was simply letting the disease run its course, accepting the loss of life in order to keep the economy open. This paradigm could be called "surrender." This approach rejected the idea that the disease was an existential threat, and proponents therefore sought to squelch any instinct to protect the population. Those who espoused this view were ready to abandon fellow citizens—the elderly and essential workers in particular.

The second paradigm could be labeled "freeze." This was a paradigm where collective stay-at-home orders were used to shut the virus down, but governments provided economic stimulus to the economy to tide it over in hopes that, once the disease had run its course, the economy could be rebooted. Businesses would restart and people would carry on as before, with the pre-pandemic economy having in a sense simply been frozen in place for some period of time. Denmark pursued this strategy most comprehensively, providing compensation to employers to avoid layoffs. Germany also undertook a version of this model. To some extent the first rounds of US stimulus were cast in this mold.

With the freeze paradigm, the expectation was that shutting the country down would "flatten the peak" and bring the reproduction rate of the virus below 1. Then society would open up for a while, but we would expect further waves to emerge, and we would expect to tighten down again. We'd expect to reintroduce stay-at-home advisories. This policy approach was characterized as using a "hard braking, slow braking" approach (Emanuel et al. 2020). If we braked hard up front, the proposal went, we could then open up but should expect several further periods of braking as we sought to decelerate the progress of the disease.

Each of these paradigms was presented as protecting either livelihoods or lives but not both. The surrender paradigm was mooted on the grounds that it was necessary to protect the economy. The freeze paradigm was mooted on the grounds that it was an expensive but necessary way of saving lives.

Yet the representation of a trade-off between lives and livelihoods in fact made no sense. The surrender paradigm, which was cast as the economy-saving paradigm, was actually the more expensive. The surrender paradigm would have led to the deaths of at least some two million people in the US, and, using conventional economists' methods for measuring the impact of a loss of life, the cost of the surrender paradigm in monetary terms was $15–20 trillion (Allen 2020). As for the freeze paradigm, it was also expensive. In April, estimates were that it would cost tens of billions of dollars a day to have the economy shut down, or roughly $350 billion a month, for a one-quarter decline of about 5 percent of GDP. It turned out we underestimated. GDP fell by 32 percent in the second quarter of 2020. Moreover, an expectation of repeated phases of stay-at-home advisories would have been a further hindrance to

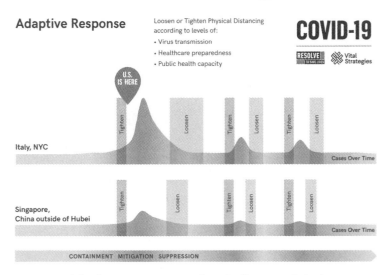

FIGURE 5. Adaptive response strategy from April 2020, early in the pandemic response

SOURCE: Prevent Epidemics 2020

economic recovery by making business planning exceptionally difficult. No full economic restart is possible when businesses face phases of opening and closing, opening and closing, with no predictable pattern. Fast economic recovery would have required knowing that we could reopen and stay open. Consequently, we needed disease control powerful enough to fend off subsequent waves of infection.

Sometimes, when a doctor gives a patient medicine, the medicine turns out to have side effects that might kill the patient. Some cancer patients, for instance, are not able to endure the prescribed course of chemotherapy. When that happens, their physicians change course. They find an alternative way of treating the disease that also preserves the underlying resources for life that that patient needs to fight the disease. Our economy is that set of resources for life that we need to fight the disease.

In fighting the pandemic, the job we faced in March and April was to recognize that the medicine we had for this pandemic also had the side effect of killing the economy. We needed an alternative.

I'll turn now to reviewing the five elements of that alternative: (1) a culture of adherence to universal precautions of mask-wearing, and hand and bathroom hygiene supportive of infection control; (2) a supply chain and implementation infrastructure to support TTSI; (3) schools safely open for in-person learning; (4) safe in-person services via screening testing; and (5) effective public communication.

Universal Precautions

The world has known plague from the earliest of times, including many prior examples of airborne respiratory diseases. East Asian nations dealt with SARS in the early 2000s and Middle Eastern nations with MERS in 2012. From biblical recommendations that lepers cover their mouths with a cloth to the twenty-first-century SARS and MERS outbreaks, a routine element of protecting against an epidemic, and especially an airborne epidemic, has involved the adherence to a basic set of universally practiced precautions, including mask-wearing and regular handwashing. This element of pandemic response policy should have been a no-brainer, particularly since it was clear from an early point that the Asian nations—which had previous experience with coronavirus and were most successfully fighting the pandemic—had made mask-wearing a foundational element of their response.

Masks reduce the likelihood of virus transmission from an infectious person to others. They have no negative effect on the economy. In fact, a sudden surge of demand for masks presents an economic opportunity for the textile industry. Finally, their impact on liberty is minimal: masks (with face shields as an alternative) hinder few people's ability to pursue their vocations, their religions, their associations, or their expression of beliefs. Nor do they impinge on civil and political liberties. They impinge no more than the requirement to wear clothing when we are out in public. Indeed, locales that require masks can be understood simply to be extending the definition of a requirement for clothing in public, justified by the need to protect others from indecent exposure.

Testing, Tracing, and Supported Isolation (TTSI)

A second tool for interrupting transmission is a package of activities now commonly known as "testing, tracing, and isolating." In this approach, diagnostic testing is used to find the virus and break its chain of transmission. All those with symptoms are tested, and those with whom they've been in contact while infectious are also tested and, for any of those contacts who test positive, their contacts are also tested. The goal is to test all the way down the chain of virus transmission and to make sure that all those who test positive isolate, that is, spend time away from contact with other people until they are no longer infectious.

The work of having those who test positive isolate, however, also requires supports for those for whom isolation is difficult. It's particularly difficult for low-income workers who are asymptomatic or presymptomatic to isolate. If they find that they test positive, they will have to give up two weeks, say, of time in the labor force, losing wages that they will surely need in order to get through the experience of isolation itself. If workers don't have paid sick leave or job protection, isolation is not really viable unless there are actual supports provided for it (Laughland and Holpuch 2020). Also, low-income workers often live in multigenerational, multiperson households, where staying away from others is in itself difficult. In New York City, the Test and Trace team found that those who tested positive, were required to isolate, lived in dense residential situations, and needed help, typically needed food, assistance securing wage replacement, and personal protective equipment to help them keep from infecting others. The policy package we needed was not "testing, tracing, and isolating" merely but "testing, tracing, and supported isolation," or TTSI (Allen, Block, et al. 2020).

Asian nations like South Korea and Taiwan provided examples of the TTSI policy framework in action. Right from the get-go, South Korean public health authorities were clear that their goal was to interrupt chains of transmission. For every positive case they found, they would trace the individuals who had been exposed to that infectious person, test those individuals, trace their contacts and test again, tracking down a whole network or chain of transmission. In one example, when South Korea did have a major outbreak, it was rapidly traced back to the gathering of a large church congregation. They then tested everybody in that congregation to find all the cases. By virtue of doing that, they were able to keep the outbreak from accelerating the disease throughout the country. Early in the pandemic, South Korea was testing twenty-five further people for every positive case they found. That level of follow-up, applied to the United States in May, would have required us to be testing five million rather than the three hundred thousand people per day that we were then managing.

Of course, that number of five million tests per day nationally would have been composed optimally of different levels of testing in different parts of the country depending on disease prevalence. That made it very hard to give a one-size-fits-all answer to the question of how any locale should suppress

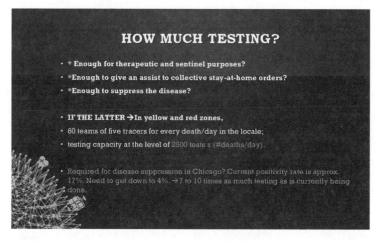

FIGURE 6. Local testing targets for a TTSI strategy

COVID-19. Local variation in how the disease unfolded meant workable policy needed to be structured from the ground up, with descriptions of how decision-making should work in specific places. Figure 6 provides an example of how the aggregate policy paradigm could have been rendered in a form useful to local decision-makers.

Success would ultimately have been dependent on the more than four thousand counties in this country, that is, on people who knew their communities and could figure out the right way to make sure that locally trusted parties were the ones responsible for these programs. Thus success at launching a TTSI program required empowering local actors—mayors and county health officials in particular—and equipping them with the tools for knowing how to set their targets, how to organize, sort, and process sample collections, how to connect the labs, access lab capacity, and so forth. Contextual tailoring was necessary for success.

Like masks, TTSI reduces occurrences of virus transmission by limiting the amount of interaction infectious people have with others. This policy approach has no negative effect on the economy. In fact, a sudden surge of demand for testing presents an economic opportunity for the biotechnology sector. The need for an exceedingly rapid ramp-up of testing, in a context where we had not yet built the infrastructure for it, did demand federal intervention to support rapid recomposition of the economy, but all this was doable in economy-strengthening ways. Nor was the necessary federal investment nearly as expensive as the costs of either the surrender or the freeze paradigm. Total supply and personnel cost of a TTSI program over twelve months would have been about $180 billion, less than one month's cost projected for the freeze paradigm.

The most significant challenge to the TTSI paradigm emerges along the liberty dimension. Requests to those who test positive for information about the people with whom they've interacted can be experienced as a violation of privacy. The requirement that those who test positive for COVID-19 isolate constitutes a restriction of liberty and mobility. These infringements of liberty, however, are well within bounds already established by the law of public health emergencies as justified by a public interest in halting a dangerous pandemic.

Indeed, shoe-leather contact tracing is a tried-and-true technique in public health and regularly in use. Every year there are outbreaks of infectious diseases in the United States that require contact tracing in order to achieve control: tuberculosis; measles; syphilis. We never pay attention because these outbreaks never turn into broad epidemics: often because contact tracing is used to find those who have been exposed and to have them quarantine until the danger of transmission passes. For all of those routine contact tracing and quarantine orders, we already have existing policy protocols for how to protect civil liberties. Patient privacy, as protected by HIPAA (Health Insurance Portability and Accountability Act), for instance, applies to contact tracing. And typically one of the legal requirements for quarantine or isolation is that there be a definite timetable. The lack of clear timetables for our collective stay-at-home orders when they were first imposed in spring 2020 was one of their most problematic features. While there was initially concern about digital contact tracing apps and privacy, it was clear early on that digital apps were unlikely to gain traction in the United States or to achieve valuable functionality; they were a nonissue by May. To the degree that they were adopted in Europe, those apps that succeeded were also the apps with the most extensive privacy protections (Leprince-Ringuet 2020). European privacy frameworks—and in particular the German framework—provided a robust foundation for the reasonable introduction of new technologies in alignment with recognizable standards of privacy protection. The policy paradigm we needed would not in fact have introduced new challenges to civil liberties.

Even more important, however, with regard to quarantine, isolation, and contact tracing, the ethical duty not to harm others generates a positive duty on the part of those who have been exposed to COVID-19 and on the part of the COVID-19-positive individual to participate in public health measures. The exposed person and the COVID-19-positive person have an obligation, respectively, to quarantine or to isolate so as not to harm others; the COVID-19-positive person has to make sure that those whom they may have exposed to the disease receive notification of that fact. Strictly speaking, neither contact tracing nor isolation require implementation by health authorities. These are both practices that we all ought to take up ourselves, recognizing them as do-it-yourself moral duties. Indeed, we might best understand contact tracing as simply a peer-to-peer warning that someone has been exposed to the virus and may be endangering others.

Importantly, in the context of a liberal democracy, a TTSI policy paradigm requires significant reserves of solidarity. We maximize the effectiveness of this set of public health tools to the degree that we cultivate a norm of not doing harm to others. Many people facing COVID-19 were willing to undertake sacrifices to protect friends and family, for instance, standing in line for hours to get a diagnostic test before seeking to visit a relative with health vulnerabilities. Solidarity extends that integration of our own good with the good of others to the full extent of our political community. Public health officials, then, have the responsibility to maximize participation in these practices, by ensuring that even those who are not in the first instance responsive to the call of duty or solidarity, or who have competing demands of necessity, are also able to participate in this prosocial activity.

Safe School Reopenings

Rapid suppression of COVID-19 in March and April through masking and TTSI would have made safe in-person learning an easy policy to pursue in September. In the absence of that suppression, however, we needed a policy framework for opening schools safely for in-person learning *despite* community spread.

As Meira Levinson and Jacob Fay have argued, spring school closures revealed what we as a society have come to see as the most essential features of schools: provision of nutrition to low-income learners and childcare for workers (Levinson and Fay 2020). When schools closed, districts everywhere had to figure out how to get meals to kids who depended on them. Similarly, school closures left workers at all socioeconomic levels scrambling to find alternative childcare arrangements; the result has been a significant withdrawal of women from the labor force (Badger 2020). This withdrawal reduces the life prospects of those women and their families as well as reducing economic productivity generally.

In other words, schools, and especially public schools, are no longer just sites for learning. They have also become critical nodes in a de facto networked structure for the provision of welfare and social services by state governments: in essence, the national safety net—providing not only food but also health resources to disadvantaged students and providing free child-care to every member of the population who chooses to use public schools. Remote schooling has been bad for learners, but it has also revealed the degree to which schools themselves are a fundamental building block of the economy in their day-to-day operations. That is, they are a fundamental building block not—as usually understood—simply because they prepare young people for the workforce. They are a fundamental building block because they are a significant safety net for the workforce.

Closing schools to in-person learning turned out to be another form of medicine intended to fight the disease but which undermines the health of the patient. Here too we needed a solution that would permit us to keep schools open for in-person learning, even with community spread. Judging the degree of risk involved for in-person learning at different levels of community spread was challenging. It was not until the early summer of 2020 that we began to have a clear picture that children transmitted COVID-19 less frequently than older adults. It was also only in the summer that we achieved confirmation of the substantially lower impacts of COVID-19 on children. But as those facts came into view, so did the elements of a strategy for safe in-person learning, even with community spread.

Schools needed to become masters of infection control, in a fashion similar to hospitals, so that they might become—among all our institutions other than hospitals—last to close and first to open for most students. For special needs students, and the youngest learners who cannot learn well remotely

(K–3), they need to be always open for in-person learning. For schools to become masters of infection control meant they needed to develop organizational capacity to establish universal precautions like mask-wearing, achieve environmental improvements to ventilation and filtration, and reorganize programs and practices to achieve physical distancing.

Here too testing, tracing, quarantine, and isolation were valuable tools that should have been put in use. In this context, the policy we needed was not one of diagnostic testing followed by contact tracing but screening testing. "Screening testing" designates routine testing of the nonsymptomatic to identify asymptomatic cases and to make sure that any cases entering the school community immediately lead both to contact tracing and to the infectious person entering isolation. Following research by the Duke-Margolis Center for Health Policy, a good target would be testing K–12 educators, paraprofessionals, staff, once a week in all contexts, while also adding in the weekly testing of high school students in contexts with high community spread (Rivers et al. 2020).

In contrast to masks and TTSI, keeping schools open for in-person learning with screening testing and new infection protocols does not reduce rates of virus transmission in the community. However, the data show that, with robust practices of infection control, schools can offer in-person learning *without increasing* local rates of transmission (Jha and Nair-Desai 2020). In-person learning can be offered safely, and doing so supports livelihoods and the economy without undermining the effort to suppress the disease itself. Safety in schools will pay rewards in the form of a healthier economy, but achieving that safety will take meaningful investment, at levels necessary to counteract decades of neglect of school buildings and properties.

While it is important to recognize schools as filling essential functions in our society, that does not necessarily mean that educators, paraprofessionals, and school staff should be designated as "essential workers." That may not be the right pathway to achieve continuity in teaching and learning in conditions of emergency. In some cases, that designation can bring hazard pay and bonuses. In other cases, however, that designation can lead to liberty-violating efforts to force people to report to work against their will. Schools offering in-person learning should be staffed on the basis of freely chosen commitments to work. Educators, paraprofessionals, and staff will participate if they can trust both that the environment in which they work is safe and that they can get to and from work safely. As with the need for solidarity in the broader society to support effective pandemic response, so too in schools trust among administrators, educators, staff, students, and families is perhaps the most critical resource needed to achieve safe in-person learning.

Safety for Businesses Requiring In-Person Interaction

A fourth piece, one largely neglected, of a successful policy framework would have addressed the gap between the impact of the COVID-19 pandemic on affluent telecommuters and on workers whose jobs depend on services requiring in-person interaction. In order to achieve recovery for the whole economy, businesses that depended on in-person interaction needed tools and resources for the infection control and safety measures necessary to restore consumer confidence.

During this pandemic, the wealthy were able to retreat to vacation homes and telecommuting lifestyles—much as ancient Romans and early modern British aristocrats used to retreat to villas and country estates in the face of plague. But those who typically provided them with services suffered. Indeed, as economists have pointed out, the COVID-19 crisis highlighted the significant dependence of ordinary workers on

Roadmap to Pandemic Resilience

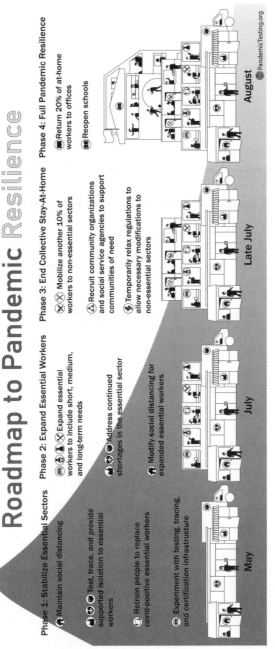

Phase 1: Stabilize Essential Sectors
- Maintain social distancing
- Test, trace, and provide supported isolation to essential workers
- Retrain people to replace covid-positive essential workers
- Experiment with testing, tracing, and certification infrastructure

May

Phase 2: Expand Essential Workers
- Expand essential workers to include short, medium, and long-term needs
- Address continued shortages in the essential sector
- Modify social distancing for expanded essential workers

July

Phase 3: End Collective Stay-At-Home
- Mobilize another 10% of workers to non-essential sectors
- Recruit community organizations and social service agencies to support communities of need
- Temporarily relax regulations to allow necessary modifications to non-essential sectors

Late July

Phase 4: Full Pandemic Resilience
- Return 20% of at-home workers to offices
- Reopen schools

August

PandemicTesting.org

FIGURE 7. From "Roadmap to Pandemic Resilience"—original proposal for reopening schedule

SOURCE: Allen, Block, et al. 2020; visual created by M Eifler

the consumption habits of the wealthy. "Households in the top 25 percent of the income distribution are responsible for over half of the overall spending reduction" (Williams et al. 2020). These affluent households particularly reduced their spending on services requiring in-person interactions: hotels, transportation, food services, barbers and beauty salons. By July employment levels for the affluent were nearly back to precrisis levels, but the shift in their patterns of consumption—away from in-person services—was durable. Consequently, "employment rates among low-wage workers [were] still down by over 15 percent through mid-September" (Williams et al. 2020). The pandemic has made visible the tale of two countries that lies beneath the structure of our economy.

Screening testing would have been valuable for businesses that depend on interpersonal interaction and should have been a higher priority than the use of screening testing for affluent workers able to telecommute (see fig. 7). Such an effort should have been the focus of policy in support of small business. For small businesses, restoring a foundation of health, and public confidence in the general public health, was the only available path toward full economic recovery.

Public Communication

The final component of a successful COVID-19 response would have been a clear and coherent program of public communication. First, there was a need to communicate the overarching goal of aligning protection of lives, livelihoods, and liberties. Second, there was a need to communicate the interdependence of individual and public health with the economy. Third, it was critical to introduce the public to new tools and concepts: massively scaled-up testing, contact tracing and supported isolation; screening testing as a complement to diagnostic testing;

in-person learning in school buildings as filling essential functions in the economy; and a need for reciprocity in support of those whose businesses and jobs were affected by the turn away from in-person services. Fourth and finally, there was a need to clarify for the public what each citizen's individual responsibilities were in order to avoid bringing harm to others and to accelerate the full return of beloved activities—from football games to church attendance.

Why We Failed to Adopt This Strategy

As noted in chapter 1, the first reaction of many commentators to the flailing response in the United States was to warn that either democracy or federalism per se was the root of the problem. But this was not the case. As I will spell out in more detail in chapter 3, the United States' tiered structure of government—with authority over public health residing in officials from the president all the way down to the county health officer—was actually an invaluable resource. It makes contextually tailored policy possible—and this is just what we needed.

For instance, as public health authorities discovered in the HIV-AIDS crisis, contact-tracing programs are most effective when they are run by people trusted within the community in which they operate. While American distrust of national government has risen continuously over the last few decades, trust in local government remains high. Relatedly, a contact-tracing program that protects privacy, for example, is best introduced at the local level. If sensitive data about everyone a person has interacted with were funneled into a centralized national database, the potential for abuse would be high. While no database is without its vulnerabilities, small pockets of data are of much less value to hackers or profiteers than nationally centralized databases. While we surely want the federal government to help design the IT infrastructure used by local health officials, for the sake of benefiting from scale, it's reasonable to leave use of that infrastructure in the hands of local authorities, subject to audit and review by the state.

We needed the federal government to focus on the big picture: to set overarching goals and identify promising practices for how best to preserve lives, livelihoods, and liberties simultaneously. Then we needed state, county, metropolitan, and municipal governments to get into the nitty-gritty: contact tracing, testing, treating the ill, and supporting those who are isolating. The institutional setup is well enough arranged to have supported that kind of response; what went wrong was a failure of governance.

As we saw in chapter 1, we found ourselves vulnerable along all of the core dimensions of democratic governance. We were not ready to carry out integrated policy-making. Our broken social contract left us with diminished stores of solidarity. And the White House did not use the country's foremost teaching platform to teach responsibly, even though public understanding and acceptance are among the most important resources for effective implementation of any policy. Yet our governance failures also reflected our own civic weaknesses as a people. While plenty of complaints and grievances were directed at President Trump and other public officials, public opinion lacked clear focus on what we needed—good governance, and the four elements of good governance discussed above.

For decades now, the American public's understanding of the demands and requirements of governance has atrophied. That point hit home for me personally after Trump was elected in 2016, when disgruntled Americans of all ages and from around the country wrote me asking how they could play a civic role and make a difference by influencing their country to lean

Doesn't make connection *Expert?*

into the values they cared about. (Evidently, being a historian of American constitutional democracy and a political philosopher of democracy was enough to mark me as a civic "Dear Abby.") What astonished me was how few people knew where to start. They did not know how to call a meeting, how to shape a conversation around diagnosis of our circumstances, or how to engage their fellow Americans in conversation about finding some sort of shared purpose.

If the previous sentence was opaque, that is an example of the problem. It would not have been opaque to the people who opened the Declaration of Independence by writing, "When in the course of human events, it becomes necessary . . ." The work of politics begins by diagnosing the course of human events. What is going well and what is going badly? And why? And on what basis do you judge that something is going well or badly? These are the questions that many Americans do not know how to engage their fellow Americans in asking and answering; these are the questions that could lead to practical decisions about how to engage with political institutions to effect change.

Constitutional democracy is simply a set of institutions that give people the chance to do these things and, if they do them well, to shape their communities. Yet Americans no longer understood how to use the machinery sitting all around them.

Instead of dwelling on critique after critique of President Trump or Speaker Pelosi, Americans might have asked themselves, What questions need to be answered here? They might have registered that public health experts have only part of the answer: they know how to fight diseases. Similarly, economists have a separate part of the answer: they know how to keep liquidity flowing or how to stimulate a sinking economy. But we needed an answer that put these parts together, in an integrated judgment about how to align the full set of our overarching objectives.

There was a spark of such a moment when President Trump said, about collective stay-at-home orders, that the cure "cannot . . . be worse than the problem itself" (Haberman and Sanger 2020). That was right. That moment was a call for proposals—a call for alternative ways of addressing the health problem that would not be economy-killing. But most of the country did not hear his remark that way. And the White House itself didn't understand the value of what had been said enough to follow up on it fully: with transparent deliberation and clear public education.

As I said above, a common purpose is not an airy-fairy thing. It is a practical tool that permits people to achieve something together. A common purpose is, in effect, a map marked with a destination, a guide that permits collaborative navigation. It is perhaps the most powerful tool in the democratic toolkit, particularly in a crisis, because it can yield the solidarity that enables people to do hard things voluntarily rather than through authoritarian compulsion. Yet the tool is disintegrating from disuse.

We must next ask why Americans' understanding of constitutional democracy and of individuals' roles within it has atrophied. The answer probably goes back to another crisis. When World War II hit, the country mobilized behind the common purpose of defeating the Axis threat. As part of that effort, the US military, intent on beating Germany in developing an atomic bomb, activated the scientific community through the Manhattan Project. That was the beginning of the scientification of American society.

After the Cold War began, and especially after the launch of Sputnik in 1957, the United States invested increasingly in research and STEM (science, technology, engineering, and math) education. The goal was to remain globally competitive in both economic and military terms. Americans were inspired afresh in 1983 by *A Nation at Risk*, the report of a federal commission, which found that the United States' "once unchallenged preeminence in commerce, industry, science, and technological innovation is being overtaken by competitors throughout the world" (National Commission on Excellence in Education 1983). More recently, the National Academy of Science's 2007 report *Rising above the Gathering Storm* worried that "that the scientific and technological building blocks critical to our economic leadership are eroding at a time when many other nations are gathering strength" (National Academy of Sciences 2007).

The United States needs science. It needs technological innovation, and it needs scientists to advise elected leaders. But this is not all that the country needs. The country also needs people who make judgment calls. At the end of the day, we have to rebuild our understanding of what judgment is as a practice, what judgment consists of, and how technical expertise advises judgment but shouldn't replace it. The humanities are a set of disciplines that I think best teach synthetic understanding and that best teach people how to consider human goals, whether individual or collective. The judgments that we need at the heart of our politics should always be with reference to the broadest human goals, not decisions as matters of technical, logistical decision-making.

The US government's growing investments in scientific education have been accompanied by reductions in funding for civic education. We downshifted from delivering three courses in civics to most high school students in the mid-twentieth century to now delivering one single-semester course to approximately 85 percent of students. Nine states have no civic education requirements. Only 23 percent of eighth graders test as proficient in civics on the NAEP (National Assessment of Educational Progress) exam. We spend roughly $50 per student per year on STEM fields and 5 cents per student per year on civics.

What's more, science education is negatively correlated with political participation: researchers have found that the more hours of science courses students take, the less likely they are to vote and partake in other aspects of civic life (Allen 2016). Over the course of nearly eight decades of investing in scientific competitiveness, the United States neglected the civic side of the equation.

And the country is paying for it now. In the United States today, the art of governance is, at best, on life support. Paradoxically, in the four years of his administration, Trump delivered the best civics lesson in generations. Thanks to his impeachment trial, Americans have had to think about the proper bounds of executive power, the checks offered by the legislative and judicial branches, and precepts of the Constitution. Thanks to his failure to govern through this crisis, many have learned for the first time just how the United States' federal system is supposed to work.

Indeed, this crisis has stripped bare the truth of the vulnerability, fragility, and unsteadiness of our constitutional democracy. We had all the public health and economic knowledge that we needed to respond to this crisis, but not the common purpose that could have given us reason to draw on that knowledge effectively. If the country's constitutional democracy is to have a healthy future, Americans should finish this crisis intending not only to invest in health infrastructure but also to revive civic education. This book seeks to show the way. In this chapter, I've tried to exemplify the kind of integrative political judgment that's necessary in a constitutional democracy. In the next chapter, I'll lay out how a strategy of collaborative federalism could have served us well over the course of this pandemic, could have supported pandemic resilience, and could still become the basis of much more effective policy-making for justice, health, and democracy going forward. Chapter 3 will both seek to revive our shared understanding of the value in our federal system and provide an innovative approach to accessing that value in the twenty-first century. Until we rebuild our understanding of our federal system, we cannot and will not use it well.

3

Federalism Is an Asset

In March 2020—which feels like a lifetime ago but is not that far behind us—the press was trumpeting a narrative about chaos in coronavirus response. The *Washington Post*, for instance, ran a story on March 24 entitled "Scramble for Medical Equipment Descends into Chaos as US States and Hospitals Compete for Supplies" (Whalen et al. 2020). On April 8, the paper ran "In the Absence of a National Testing Strategy, States Go Their Own Way" (Eilperin et al. 2020). The Trump administration responded to that media narrative by arguing that it did in fact have a national strategy, namely, decentralization and federalism. Supportive publications celebrated a policy-making breakthrough. On April 17, the *Wall Street Journal* reported: "Trump Rewrites the Book on Emergencies: For the First Time in US History an Administration Is Responding to Crisis with Deregulation and Decentralization" (DeMuth 2020). On May 8, the *Federalist* proclaimed, "Trump's Federalist Approach to the Virus Is Working" (Marcus 2020).

In fact, Trump's federalist approach did not work, not because of a lack of validity as a policy path but because of a lack of steadiness, seriousness, and follow-through. The pathway proposed could have worked and, in the administration's hamfisted efforts to shift responsibility and potential blame for weaknesses in coronavirus response to governors, the Trump team accidentally revealed one of our most valuable assets—our multilayered federal system—and gave us a tantalizing glimpse of how it could be put to work for us, if we put our minds to the task for real.

Federalism *is* an asset. In other parts of the world, the pandemic has been most easily controlled in population units smaller than massive nations such as the United States. China controlled the pandemic by locking down Wuhan specifically. Singapore, Hong Kong, Taiwan, Iceland, New Zealand, and Australia have been able to draw on properties of their island status and smaller populations to fend off the virus. By early April, Iceland, with a population of just over three hundred thousand, had tested 10 percent of its population; the small town of Vò, Italy, had tested everybody. The network properties of virus transmission mean that controls aligned to the existing networked structure of social life perform better than those disconnected from those networked structures. A case study is the contrast between Singapore and South Korea. After early success in suppressing the virus, Singapore saw a widespread outbreak which originated from a failure to control the virus within its migrant community; in other words, it overlooked a dense node of social relations in a marginalized community. South Korea, in contrast, moved swiftly at key points to control spread within specific communities and social networks— early on, a large church congregation, and, at another important point, social communities frequenting a specific set of bars and nightclubs (Mokhtar 2020). The best way of aligning COVID-19 response to the properties of disease transmission is to lodge authority for key public health decisions at the level of state and local authorities who are best positioned to understand and respond to the dynamics of community spread.

Simultaneously, however, those state and local authorities

need conditions for success. The island nations combine an ability to make policy at levels closely tied to social network structures with the ability to achieve full coordination of a national economy in support of that policy. Because of our tiered structure, public health authorities at the state and local level are without one of the tools they need—economic coordination at the national level. For this, they need leadership and support from the upper tier, the federal government.

Our tiered structure is valuable because it modularizes our society and makes it possible to deploy policy programs on smaller scales in context-specific ways. Contact tracing with privacy protection is a clear example of both the benefits of a tiered federal system and of the dependence of those benefits on actors within the system performing their proper roles. If contact-tracing programs that depend on highly sensitive data are anchored at the local level, rather than flowing into nationally centralized databases, they don't pose the same degree of threat to civil liberties or introduce the same capacity for governmental surveillance and control. While that tiering of our federal structure and situating of policy authority at lower levels provides resilience and protection, success also requires support from the upper tiers of the system.

But to see the value of federalism for the crisis at hand is not necessarily to concur that the White House has successfully led a federalist strategy. To evaluate that question, we have to look more deeply into federalism itself, its history and key principles.

In what follows, I take a close look at American federalism, outlining key elements of the federalist framework developed both at the time the Constitution was written and during a period of twentieth-century renovation. I lay out the value of an innovative "collaborative federalism" for our own moment and offer a brief evaluation of whether the White House achieved a genuinely federalist strategy.

Key Features of the Federalist Framework

The problem we faced in March and April was very similar to that in the period between the American Revolution and the Constitutional Convention—but in reverse.

Then, the national government needed revenue to handle war debts and ongoing obligations for which it had responsibility, yet it had no authority to secure those revenues from the states. Instead, it was at the mercy of states' autonomous decisions about whether to hand over revenue to the federal government. Fully masters of their own revenue, states simultaneously set up tariffs among themselves with the result that interstate commerce was breaking down.

Now, in 2020 the states had responsibility for delivering boots-on-the-ground coronavirus response, but had neither the fiscal capacity nor the organizational authority to recompose the economy to deliver the matter and matériel needed—tests and other supplies—to suppress COVID-19. They needed the federal government to secure those resources on their behalf, even as they took responsibility for implementation of a public health response. Yet the federal government was not delivering.

A fundamental purpose of the drafting of the US Constitution was to achieve an alignment of responsibilities and authorities for federal and state governments such that the system as a whole could function to deliver safety and happiness to the people. This point was made in the *Federalist Papers*, the essays written by Alexander Hamilton, James Madison, and John Jay in defense of the new Constitution. *Federalist* no. 43, written by Madison, took up the question of why the drafters of the Constitution had settled on a process by which a supermajority of nine states, rather than full unanimity, would suffice to ratify the Constitution. Madison wrote (emphasis added):

On what principle [can] the Confederation, which stands in the solemn form of a compact among the States, . . . be superseded without the unanimous consent of the parties to it?. . . . The first question is answered at once by recurring to the absolute necessity of the case; to the great principle of self-preservation; to the transcendent law of nature and of nature's God, *which declares that the safety and happiness of society are the objects at which all political institutions aim, and to which all such institutions must be sacrificed.*

In invoking the law of nature and of nature's God as well as the safety and happiness of the people, both phrases from the Declaration of Independence, Madison was tying the Constitution back to the Declaration and its assertion that the purpose of political institutions was to deliver the safety and happiness of the people. As I mentioned earlier, that phrase, "safety and happiness," was a late eighteenth-century translation of the Roman phrase *Salus populi suprema lex esto*: "Let the health of the people be the supreme law." The entire purpose of our constitutional structure is to deliver *salus populi*, the health and well-being of the people, or the general welfare. The purpose of federalism itself, then, is also no less than this. But how is federalism supposed to deliver?

Tomes have been written on US federalism, starting with the *Federalist Papers*. The key characteristics of our federal system have been much debated in both their meaning and import, but five are particularly important for understanding our current moment. They are as follows:

- A tiering of responsibilities and authorities
- Federal responsibility to maintain proper harmony and intercourse among the states

- The primacy of the legislative branch
- Federal responsibility for equal protection of the laws
- Devolution of power

The drafters of the Constitution self-consciously *tiered responsibilities and authorities,* recognizing that different kinds of functionality should be handled either nationally and centrally or at a more local level, closer to the diversity of facts on the ground. They thought explicitly about the joints connecting the whole federal system and charged the national government with *maintenance of harmony and proper intercourse among the states.* Finally, they considered the legislative branch, not the executive branch, to be the first branch of government. While power has swung to the executive branch over the course of our history, and particularly over the course of the twentieth century from the Great Depression onward, it is nonetheless the case that the structure of our Constitution and federal system depend in important ways on the *primacy of the legislature.* Modernized federalism, a child of twentieth-century jurisprudence, introduces two additional key elements of particular relevance to us now: the role of the US government in guaranteeing *equal protection of the laws* for all, thereby requiring all states to adhere to protection of constitutional rights, and the recognition that in the context of demographic diversity, *devolution of power*, where possible, provides an avenue to empowering minority subpopulations (Gerken 2020). I will take each of these features in turn. These five features of our federal system are what unlocks its value.

Tiered Responsibilities and Authorities

The drafters of the US Constitution sought to establish a framework for the exercise of power that prevents its abuse. A key feature of the design was "separation of powers." Conventionally, we focus on the division of power among legislative, executive, and judicial powers and the assignment of these separable powers to different office holders and branches of government. We typically take both separation of powers and checks and balances to name the structure of operations among these three branches of government.

Yet the drafters of the US Constitution in fact extended the separation of powers approach even beyond the specific division among legislative, executive, and judicial powers. They also saw the structure of federal and state governments as a form of separation of power. Thus, either James Madison or Alexander Hamilton wrote in *Federalist* no. 51:

> In a single republic, all the power surrendered by the people is submitted to the administration of a single government; and the usurpations are guarded against by a division of the government into distinct and separate departments. In the compound republic of America, the power surrendered by the people is first divided between two distinct governments, and then the portion allotted to each subdivided among distinct and separate departments. Hence a double security arises to the rights of the people. The different governments will control each other, at the same time that each will be controlled by itself.

Finally, they also recognized different substantive domains of policy as creating distinct channels of power, and they separated substantive policy domains in order to drive the exercise of power into separable channels. The assignment of some substantive powers to the federal government and some to state governments further functioned to separate powers for the sake of reining in likely abuses. Hamilton sketched the point in broad strokes in *Federalist* no. 17; it is worth reviewing his argument at length:

> It may be said that [the new Constitution] would tend to render the government of the Union too powerful, and to enable it to absorb those residuary authorities, which it might be judged proper to leave with the States for local purposes. Allowing the utmost latitude to the love of power which any reasonable man can require, I confess I am at a loss to discover what temptation the persons intrusted with the administration of the general government could ever feel to divest the States of the authorities of that description. The regulation of the mere domestic police of a State appears to me to hold out slender allurements to ambition. Commerce, finance, negotiation, and war seem to comprehend all the objects which have charms for minds governed by that passion; and all the powers necessary to those objects ought, in the first instance, to be lodged in the national depository. The administration of private justice between the citizens of the same State, the supervision of agriculture and of other concerns of a similar nature, all those things, in short, which are proper to be provided for by local legislation, can never be desirable cares of a general jurisdiction. It is therefore improbable that there should exist a disposition in the federal councils to usurp the powers with which they are connected; because the attempt to exercise those powers would be as troublesome as it would be nugatory; and the possession of them, for that reason, would contribute nothing to the dignity, to the importance, or to the splendor of the national government.

The core of Hamilton's argument was that the drafters of the Constitution had taken care to deposit with the federal government those substantive domains of policy most likely to attract the attention of hungry power-seekers, with the result that fewer areas of policy would be drawn into the worst competitions for power than would be the case in a fully centralized regime. The relevant powers of the federal government were the substantive domains of commerce, finance, negotiation, and war. Power was divided and shared among the three branches to channel competition over these fiercely sought domains of control. But other substantive domains were left to the states—justice and agriculture explicitly in this essay, and others implicitly. Health and education are two of the other critical domains eventually explicitly allocated to the states. The underlying concept of tiered functionality and responsibility was formalized in the Tenth Amendment which reads: "The powers not delegated to the United States by the Constitution, nor prohibited by it to the states, are reserved to the states respectively, or to the people."

On the basis of this Tenth Amendment, most public health authorities lie with state governments; only to the degree that public health is connected to matters of national security, interstate commerce, or the regulation of external borders are federal authorities relevant. While states have authority over internal borders, the federal interstate commerce authority does also give the federal government some authority over internal borders. In short, public health law in America is complex because authority is divided among federal, state, and local governments, necessitating a high level of coordination.[1] As a public health official in Illinois put it to me in the spring of 2020, "If you've seen one state public health system, you've seen one state public health system."

1. I suggest that readers interested in questions of legality further turn to federal, state, and local laws and regulations and to the Model State Emergency Health Powers Act.

To use our federal structure effectively, this intricacy needs to be visible to us and be understood as legitimate; hence the importance of sketching it out and reviewing its original justifications.

Maintenance of Harmony and Proper Intercourse among States

A second key feature of federalism is the role of the national government in harmonizing the activities of the states. In *Federalist* no. 41, James Madison also took up the subject of the tiered assignment of responsibility and provided the following enumeration of the powers conferred on the government of the Union:

1. Security against foreign danger;
2. Regulation of the intercourse with foreign nations;
3. Maintenance of harmony and proper intercourse among the States;
4. Certain miscellaneous objects of general utility;
5. Restraint of the States from certain injurious acts;
6. Provisions for giving due efficacy to all these powers.

The disharmony among the States that followed the introduction of the Articles of Confederation and that ultimately gave rise to the Constitutional Convention lies behind the third goal on the list: maintenance of harmony and proper intercourse among the States.

Although the delegates to the Continental Congress began work on the Articles of Confederation simultaneously with their drafting of the Declaration of Independence in the summer of 1776, they were not able to achieve ratification until March 1781. By the time the Articles were ratified, the document's authority was tenuous, with voices already raised for a revision. The challenges of financing the war had quickly brought a number of economic and political issues to a head and surfaced the weaknesses of the Articles' institutional design.

The core of the problem was that the Articles of Confederation gave the federal government no independent source of revenue. Congress and General George Washington, at the head of the army, had to rely on contributions from the states. Yet states, too, were ineffective in raising taxes and inconsistent in paying their contributions to the confederation. The government's basic ability to pay and feed its army and to raise supplies for the war effort was in question throughout the war. Moreover, trade deficits generated a shortage of specie (gold and silver), which spurred states to increase their printing of paper money, thereby driving runaway inflation: "The amount of flour that one hundred pounds in paper currency could buy dropped from 143.3 hundredweight in 1776 to 83.8 in 1777, 63.2 in 1778, 6.67 in 1779, 1.15 in 1780, and .71 in 1781" (Doerflinger 1986, 200). The economic challenges affected the war effort and political stability, of course, but also commercial activity and the prospect of domestic prosperity. As Silas Deane wrote to Declaration signer and Philadelphian James Wilson in 1780, Congress's "chronic inability to put its financial affairs in order had . . . shaken all faith in the integrity and character of America" (Smith 1956, 141).

Like Alexander Hamilton, Wilson was very concerned by this state of affairs. A Scots American well read in Scottish political economy, Wilson sought to help the young country develop a banking system to secure public credit.[2] Shortly after the loss of Charleston, South Carolina, to the British in May

2. The account that follows comes from Allen and Sneff 2019.

1780, Wilson, Thomas Willing, and Robert Morris rolled out a plan for the Bank of Pennsylvania. In July, the bank opened its doors, almost fully subscribed, with both subscribers and bank committing that all funds taken in by the bank would support the war effort. The bank was relevant not merely as a provider of capital; its backers saw it as an instrument for improving fiscal policy generally. In the Pennsylvania Assembly in November 1780, Wilson argued for the introduction of three taxes: a tax on real and personal estates, an import tax, and an excise tax. These, Wilson argued, would enable Pennsylvania to pay its war debt, and now there was a bank that could put such revenue to work in the economy. The assembly rejected Wilson's arguments, but they offer a window into early arguments about how best to secure the national public revenue necessary to stabilize the new government while also protecting popular sovereignty.

Immediately upon the heels of erecting the Bank of Pennsylvania, Wilson, Morris, Hamilton, and others turned toward building the Bank of North America. Robert Morris, the superintendent of finance for the United States, submitted a plan in 1781, and Congress approved it quickly, chartering the bank formally in December, a few months after the short-lived Bank of Pennsylvania had closed. Aiming to shore up the finances of the thirteen-state confederation, leading politicians moved quickly to link up the Bank of North America and the tax system in the states.

The effort to shore up national finances with a national bank and its bank notes introduced further stresses. The benefits accrued largely to the merchant class on the coasts. As coastal merchants sought repayment of debts from farmers, who themselves still had insufficient access to currency, the economic challenges polarized the political community. The more radical western farmers became powerful antagonists of the bank, instigating a set of dynamics that would lead eventually to the Paper Money Riot in New Hampshire in 1786 and to Shay's Rebellion in Massachusetts in 1786–87. In addition, the efforts of each state to raise funds on its own behalf as part of the effort to deal with war debt was leading to a tariff war among them. The provisions of the Articles of Confederation intended to forestall such a thing were giving way to the press of necessity.

The congressional record for January through March 1783, just before the signing of the Paris Treaty, reveals a set of extraordinary debates about the finances of the new nation and their great instability. As members of Congress tried to find revenue and to determine which creditors to pay—soldiers or states that had incurred expenses for the war—their arguments previewed those that would define the Constitutional Convention four years later. How could states that were geographically more distant from Congress and thus had not been able to tap into the public coffers during the war receive fair recompense? Of course, none could be compensated if none had contributed. This generated another set of questions. How should the responsibility to fill the national purse be allocated? Should there be an assessment of the value of the land in each state as a way of measuring what each should contribute? Should state populations be counted? If so, how should enslaved people be treated? What authority did the national government have anyway to draw tax revenue from the states?

By the summer of 1785, Congress was not functioning effectively. Frequently it had too few delegates for a quorum, and the debates continued over the financial difficulties. After the 1783 taxation debates, matters had grown still trickier. The Federalists kept the issue of amending the Articles of Confederation on the agenda, recognizing the linkages among war debt, the challenges of political economy, and the polity's institutional structure. The possibility of amending the Articles was mooted in Congress in early 1783, but, by September 1783, the anti-Federalists had gained the upper hand and the issue was tabled. As 1783 came to a close, Federalist frustration with the turn of public opinion against them led to an intensified campaign of pamphlets, letters, and newspaper articles calling for a national bank and a constitutional convention. Their adversaries also intensified the battle. In March 1785, for instance, radicals secured passage in the Pennsylvania Assembly of a law "authorizing issuance of bills of credit" to be printed on paper, and "at this news the Bank of North America responded that it was not inclined to receive such irresponsible paper" (Smith 1956, 140). The bank's adversaries began advocating revocation of its charter. When the bank's charter was revoked, it upended public confidence in the bank and even its near-term viability.

This in turn precipitated an agreement among nine states to meet in Annapolis in September 1786 to debate the question whether to hold a constitutional convention. The result, of course, was the Constitutional Convention itself and then the US Constitution. The document that organizes the powers of the US government was fundamentally motivated by a need to resolve disharmony among the states, particularly as it was emanating from a tariff war and financial and fiscal failures. The project of resolving disharmony involved aligning responsibilities and authorities. If the national government was to have responsibility for war debts, it also needed the authority to raise revenue. That issue—of the alignment of responsibility and authority—is at the crux of whether a federalist system is well organized and can operate effectively.

When the COVID-19 pandemic hit in the winter of 2020, it was not long before a similar kind of disharmony existed. States competed for the supplies and personnel necessary to meet the exigencies of the moment, and municipal and state budgets soon teetered on the brink of failure.

The economic impacts of COVID-19 can be usefully partitioned into two categories: composition effects and scale effects. Composition effects refer to collapses in the demand for certain goods and services even as demand for others is sharply rising, while scale effects refer to the aggregate size of the economy with respect to employment and output. These different categories of effects require different policy responses: redeployment at scale to deal with composition effects, and social support and financing to deal with scale effects. However, our overriding goal should have been clear. We needed to maximize the speed and aggressiveness of compositional transitions to minimize the necessity of scaling down.

A system in which states are competitors for scarce emergency goods on an unusually compressed time scale ran the risk of failing to deliver the compositional shifts necessary to fight COVID-19 successfully and also of fracturing the federal structure (in a manner similar to the colonial tariff war). Occasioned by the sudden pandemic, these problems, then, gave the federal government two jobs to do in order to maintain harmony and proper intercourse among the states: (1) temporarily control the supply chain for the resources needed to fight the pandemic; and (2) backstop state and local government fiscal health. On both fronts, the federal government was responsible, in essence, for enabling the federal system as a whole to activate and deploy surge capacity efficiently across the whole of the system. Our standing military, for instance, provides surge capacity needed for national defense, such that it can be activated to any state that needs it, even though states also have their own contingents of National Guard reserves. While the states individually maintain some surge capacity, the efficacy of national surge capacity depends on our ability to tap into resources across states in a coordinated fashion in order to allocate resources where they are most needed, and to fill gaps in those resources with federal backstops.

These issues of the supply chain and the fiscal solvency of the system as a whole were of central concern to the drafters of the Constitution in their original design. Our federalist structure is designed specifically to help on these two fronts and is appropriately activated to these ends.

Primacy of the Legislature

Recognition of the key responsibilities of the federal government to support surge capacity and coordination among states in times of national emergency does not mean that all responsibility and authority for that lies with the president. A third element of our federalist system that was salient in this crisis—though often overlooked—is the primacy of the legislative branch.

In popular understanding, the executive has become the first branch. This is perhaps best captured in an Annenberg poll about civic understanding (see fig. 8). The poll reports that only 26 percent of Americans can name the branches of government, which it then lists as "executive, judicial, and legislative." Even more important than the stunning fact of how few Americans can name all three branches is how the list itself manifests a fundamental failure of civic knowledge. In listing the executive branch first and the legislative branch last, the poll write-up makes a basic mistake about the structure of our government. Article 1 of the Constitution is devoted to legislative powers. Contrary to popular understanding, Congress is the first branch. While the poll listing captures our contemporary perception of the relative importance of the three branches of government, this was not the intended design.

The exercise of power originates with the expression of a will or intention. Congress expresses the will of the people. Hence

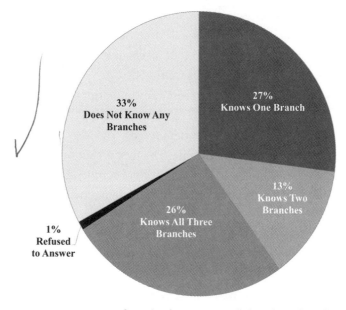

FIGURE 8. Percentage of people who can name all three branches of American government
    SOURCE: Annenberg Public Policy Center 2017

its placement in Article 1 of the Constitution. Only after the will is expressed can there be execution of the desired action. The executive branch, described in Article 2 of the Constitution, is the second branch. Judiciary comes third as a necessary mediator for addressing conflicts between the first and second branches, "the willing" and "the executing" parts of government. Nor were the three branches of government understood by the founders even as coequal, despite common parlance now.[3] In the *Federalist Papers*, the founders used the language of "coequal" institutions to refer to the taxing powers of the

3. For example, Pelosi 2019: "The genius of the Constitution, a separation of powers: three co-equal branches of government to be a check and balance on each other."

states and of the national government. They also described the House and the Senate as coequal.[4] But they did not describe the three branches of government as coequal. The legislative branch had primacy in all their writings.

Why does the degree of Congress's power matter to our collective well-being? Answering this requires revisiting the basics of the institutional design of our democracy. Two key ideas have made the American system stable. The first is that representation could be used to build a constitutional democracy at scale. The second is that durable constitutional democracies require minority-protecting mechanisms to glue electoral majorities and minorities together. The combination of popular representation, which gives power to electoral majorities, and minority-protecting mechanisms, which are a counterweight to that majority power, stabilizes our system. Each taken on its own would drive our politics into divisive conflict. These two mechanisms need to work together.

Where does popular representation actually operate in the federal government? Of the three branches, only one—Congress—carries that burden. The people speak through Congress, not through the Supreme Court, and not through the presidency, despite our massive collective hysteria about presidential elections.

Voted for by only a portion of the people, any president may choose to try to speak for the whole people—both for those affiliated with the electoral majority and also for those affiliated with the electoral minority— but nothing makes that structurally necessary. Whether the president chooses to try to represent all of us is only ever a matter of the president's character, of whether the president is moved by the better angels of his or her nature. Only Congress carries forward, as a matter of

---

4. There are seven instances of the term "coequal" in the *Federalist Papers*, including in nos. 20, 32, 34, 39, 63, and 71.

structural necessity, the voices of all the people—those in an electoral minority as well as those in the power-wielding electoral majority. Congress's job is to synthesize those voices.

Congress's primacy was clear in the Constitution but has eroded over time. An example of the shift can be found in the assignment to Congress by the Constitution of the responsibility to declare war. Over the course of the evolution of our Constitution, the president's authority to use unilateral force outside our borders has increased considerably. Initially the president's role was to *execute* war as commander-in-chief, but this soon expanded from a basis in the need to "repel sudden attacks" (1789) to the view that the president can use limited force around the globe when there is national interest in regional stability and in maintaining United Nations credibility (2011), to avert humanitarian catastrophe or to deter use of chemical weapons (2017). The reality now is that in many areas of policy where the legislative branch was intended to have primacy, the executive branch has in fact assumed it. Nonetheless, Congress's past acquiescence in the reduction of its powers does not mean it needs to rest content with the contemporary status quo. It has the power to set strategic direction.

Rather than look to the president to set strategic direction, we might look to Congress to do so. While the president has the responsibility for *executing* a national pandemic strategy, the president shares power with Congress in *setting* a pandemic strategy. Indeed, Congress's authority to declare war, and in that regard to establish overarching strategic objectives for the nation, even with regard to matters of national security, underscores the scope of Congress's powers also in the context of a pandemic. Here too Congress could and should have asserted its powers as the first branch to establish overarching strategic objectives and to appropriate funds in support of them, assigning to the president the execution of the strategy.

Those three features of federalism—tiered authorities, the goal of harmonization, and the primacy of the legislature—are three gifts from the founding era to our own that provided resources to address this pandemic as well as future challenges in the domains of health, justice, and education—domains for which state policy provides the center of gravity.

Twentieth-Century Renovations

Then twentieth-century renovations to federalism gifted us with two more critical features: the role of the US government in guaranteeing *equal protection of the laws* for all, thereby requiring all states to adhere to protection of constitutional rights; and the recognition that in the context of demographic diversity, *devolution of power* where possible provides an avenue to empowering minority subpopulations.

Equal Protection of the Laws

Madison's enumerations of the key responsibilities and authorities of the federal government included "restraint of the States from certain injurious acts." This element of federal authority was formalized in the Constitution, among other ways, in Article 4, which declared: "The United States shall guarantee to every State in this Union a Republican Form of Government." While crafted as a guarantee to states of protection from destabilization, this provision is also an effective guarantee to citizens of the right to participate in free and equal self-government.

The issue of enslavement and the question of how voting rights were determined meant that in the late eighteenth and first half of the nineteenth centuries, however, the Constitution did not in fact restrain states from acts that we would now clearly consider injurious. Indeed, the role of the federal government in restraining the states from certain injurious acts did not begin its full development until the passage of the Thirteenth, Fourteenth, and Fifteenth Amendments in the wake of the Civil War. These amendments brought protections to formerly enslaved African Americans and to working-class men, whose right to vote was now fully protected. The federal role in restraining states from injurious actions undermining the access of their citizens to participation in a republic was further extended with the dismantling of the segregationist regime established in the wake of the 1876 Hayes-Tilden agreement. *Brown v. Board of Education* (1954) and the 1964 Civil Rights Act, among other acts of jurisprudence and legislation, gave fuller definition to the Fourteenth Amendment's requirement that the federal government guarantee equal protection of the laws to all, including providing protection of constitutional rights from infringements by states.

In other words, the jurisprudence flowing from the Fourteenth Amendment has established the federal government as a bulwark of civil rights and civil liberties against state actions that might undermine them. Consequently, state governments now exercise their powers and authorities very much constrained by the requirement to deliver equal protection of the laws in relation to all the rights encoded in the Constitution. As legal scholar Heather Gerken points out, "Ours is not your father's federalism. Today's federalism is sheared of sovereignty. . . . States cannot shield their discrimination from national norms, as they did during the days of Jim Crow. If the national government wants to enforce equality norms, it can, provided it's willing to spend the political capital to do so" (Gerken 2020).

This feature of our federal system, interestingly, means that all state policies must be designed in relation to requirements of the equal protection clause. This makes state-level policy-making a valuable asset for experimenting with policy decisions to find those that best align with protection of civil rights and civil liberties.

Devolution of Power

In her writings, Gerken also highlights another feature of modernized federalism—the fifth feature of federalism under discussion here—namely the fact that the plethora of jurisdictions across our polity can be a resource for empowerment and equality (see, e.g., Gerken 2020). People who are members of minority populations within a national population can nonetheless exercise majoritarian power within more local jurisdictions, acquiring autonomy and deploying power to shape policy in ways that maximally recognize the distinctive features of their experience and perspective. As Gerken points out, this flexibility of federalism and its provision of opportunities for empowerment provides an additional route to justice. Policy can be adjusted to place and context by local decision-making and thereby more fully empower a diverse population in equitable ways. In such a policy-making context, local decision-makers can be given design principles and then asked to deliver the version of a policy for their context that best meets the objectives of these design principles. Devolution of power provides an opportunity to integrate protection of pluralism and egalitarian empowerment, a key aspect of legitimate democratic governance in the twenty-first century.

A Role for Each Part

How can these five features of federalism (tiered authorities, responsibility to maintain harmony among the states, the primacy of the legislative branch, equal protection, and devolution) guide us now, in the context of pandemic response and postpandemic recovery?

Recent Supreme Court jurisprudence has imposed limits on the ability of the federal government to compel the states to act. The court, for instance, has prohibited commandeering, whereby the federal government compels state officials to act. The court has also limited the federal government's ability to condition federal funding on state action. The federal government can nonetheless engage state governments in support of a whole-government response to an issue. The dominant approach is "cooperative federalism" in which states are given the opportunity to develop policy in particular areas (e.g., environmental regulation) against a backdrop in which the federal government, in the absence of state action, would itself directly regulate the actions of individuals and civic organizations. This pathway gives states the opportunity to tailor a broad policy framework designed in general terms by the national government to the specific needs of their state. This would have been the right approach to federalism for this crisis, had it been fully activated, because it permits quicker, more rapidly scalable action.

In addition to providing surge capacity to complement state efforts and coordinating supply chains, then, the federal government also has the responsibility to define what is a minimum acceptable "floor" for something like national security-related health policy. It is the responsibility of the federal government to ensure that the choices made by one state do not threaten public health in another state. To facilitate state autonomy and achieve the benefits of federalism while preserving a threshold foundation for public health, the federal government should have created or defined a minimally acceptable COVID-19 testing program to complement state efforts. The virtue of a system with a federally managed minimum but an emphasis on state leadership whenever possible is that it allows for the experimentation we value in our federalist system. The federal government could also utilize the federally qualified health centers, which already provide primary care to underserved populations, to provide concrete examples of the floor it seeks to establish.

Citizens should expect the federal government to set goals and targets, to identify best practices for public health, and also to establish a floor below which none will fall. They should expect their state, territorial, tribal, county, metropolitan, and municipal governments to develop and share pandemic response implementation plans.[5] Those pandemic implementation plans should include strategies for management of health care for the ill, administration of massive-scale TTSI, vaccination drives, and programs of infection control in schools. At the same time, however, citizens should also expect the federal government to secure the conditions of success for state and local actors.

Ours is a big, geographically dispersed, and geographically fragmented country with great variation in the nature of our population centers. Some places have high population density; some have low density. Up through April 2020, some parts of the country had almost no virus presence. They really should have been under different policy regimes from the hard-hit locales. The combination of local variation in circumstance and the lack of internal borders gave us a distinctively challenging situation to manage. Those features made it all the more important to deliver an aggressive surge of public health effort to eliminate the virus. Given our open internal borders,

---

5. The jurisdictional unit that should create a pandemic plan can really get quite local. See the fine examples from Eastport, Maine, and Ajo, Arizona, as described by Deborah Fallows in the *Atlantic* (Fallows 2020).

we were bound to struggle to keep the virus contained unless we truly eradicated it early and responded with equivalent speed and power to every single further outbreak. In order to deliver that kind of speed and power in responding to the virus, a key federal role in coordination was necessary, even as states brought knowledge of local circumstance to bear in maximizing the efficiency and effectiveness of response.

This review of federalism and its five features provides us with all the material we need for an ideal sketch of what a well-conceived federalist strategy might have looked like in face of a pandemic. It should have had these roles for the different parts: The federal government should have:

1. Provided surge capacity in support of health infrastructure;
2. Established a Pandemic Testing Supply Board (modeled on the War Production Board) to organize the testing supply chain (in 2021, the Biden administration acted on this via executive order);
3. Provided consistent and reliable scientific and policy guidance to states from the Department of Health and Human Services and CDC, supported by the National Academy of Sciences;
4. Conducted national "disease surveillance," for monitoring disease outbreaks and trajectories;
5. Maintained liquidity and fiscal viability in the system as a whole; and
6. Maintained safety-net testing and contact-tracing programs in communities that are not being effectively served by their state, tribal, and local governments.

State governments should have:

1. Activated state and national public health infrastructure surge capacity;

2. Established design principles for county and municipal-level social distancing, travel restriction, and pandemic testing programs, fully integrating alignment with public health standards and ethics (see Public Health Leadership Society 2002), equal protection standards, due process, nondiscrimination standards, civil liberties, privacy protections, and labor protection standards;[6]
3. Established design principles for safe in-person learning;
4. Backstopped access to personnel and supply resources for all counties, municipalities, and tribal governments to administer testing and tracing programs to target levels;
5. Worked to coordinate efforts among counties, municipalities, and tribal governments;
6. Coordinated with neighboring states, especially where it is common for individuals to live in one state but work in another; and
7. Provided universal, free access to testing and subsequent necessary medical treatment for COVID-19-positive individuals without insurance.

Tribal authorities and county, metropolitan, municipal, and regional authorities should have:

1. Deployed public health surge capacity in support of treatment of the ill and provision of support to the isolated;

---

6. These design principles, in other words, should deliver to localities parameters for their choices that are in alignment with the pertinent legal structures; localities would not themselves answer the complex legal questions involved in this space, but rather would make a set of implementation choices within frameworks developed by the state. Ideally, the American Law Institute would develop a "model law" that states could use to develop their own basic framework for a testing program.

2. Designed and administered pandemic testing and tracing programs for their communities in accordance with the standards set by the state;

3. Recorded and reported pandemic relevant data upward to state and national public health laboratories in support of ongoing disease surveillance.

As it happens, our state, county, municipal, and tribal governments often took on many of the tasks outlined above. Watching them swing into gear to get this work done was rewarding and moving. The weak link in our federal system was the national government, which failed to meet all of the responsibilities both aligned with its authorities and necessary to deliver to states the supports they needed for success.

The Weak Link in the Chain

Federalism is not, as is commonly believed, simply about handing over responsibility to the states. It is instead about activating each level of our federal system for fulfillment of its proper roles and responsibilities. Here it is worth pausing on what the word "federal" actually means. It comes, of course, from the Latin word *foedus*, meaning "treaty" or "compact." And *foedus* itself comes from *fides*, meaning trust or faith. A federal compact is about the ties binding parts to one another, not about their separation from one another. In the context of US federalism, the national government has the job of activating the ties that bind fifty states and eleven territories in support of a coordinated, harmonized, but tiered national strategy. This did not occur. The Trump administration failed to understand and activate the most valuable aspects of federalism.

Let's take the issue of mask-wearing as an example for how harmonization could have been brought about. The public education element of governance is itself complicated in a federalist context. If successful public education is coming from the White House, that takes a burden away from governors, for example. But in the absence of that, then fifty different platforms of public education result in a lot of inconsistency and conflict. It's much harder to develop and build a coherent national conversation. In the academy we are used to a competition of ideas, but in the midst of crisis, it was important that one idea win, and that the public education conducted by the federal administration align and harmonize with public education being conducted by state governments. In a moment of crisis, we needed to prioritize coordination and cooperation over competition. In the absence of a coordinating White House, to the degree that governors coordinated with other governors and began to develop shared messages and shared approaches, we helped ourselves, but even such effort could not overcome the lack of consistent messaging from the White House.

Has federalism come to fruition anywhere in action against this pandemic? Indeed, it has. As mentioned in chapter 1, Germany and Australia are places that get credit for making federalism work in the early crisis phases of the pandemic. Here is one example of harmonization in action. When the pandemic hit in Germany, one of the first things the national government did was direct resources to local health authorities to upgrade their IT systems so that the entire country could function with common data systems for tracking the disease and suppression activities. The national government relied on state and local decision-making, but it equipped everybody with the same tools, the same vocabulary, the same metrics framework so they could be part of the same conversation and act with common purpose. That was an excellent model of success.

How does a tiered system get corrected when it's not working as well as it should? The benefit of democracy and a democratic system of governance is that civil society is also a real part of the structure. It's the responsibility of individuals and organizations in a civil society to understand that tiered structure and to be able to advocate on behalf of its functioning. A lot of good efforts are underway to make things work effectively. We can point to governors; we can point to how states have formed regional compacts and coordinating bodies to move the work of pandemic response forward. Governor Larry Hogan of Maryland pulled together a network of some twenty states to address the supply-chain issues left unattended by the national government. We can point to the many civil society nonprofits, from the Rockefeller Foundation to a variety of universities and think tanks, that have supported governors in this work.

What can tie the levels of our federal system together? A common purpose. At the most basic level, the question whether our response to COVID-19 should be a strategy of therapy for the ill, mitigation of the disease, or full elimination was never resolved in the spring and summer of 2020. This returns me to the subject of chapter 1: governance.

A sixth feature of federalism that is central to its success is governance: the setting of a national strategy that successfully activates a healthy social contract, that clarifies the complementary and mutually supportive roles of each layer of our system, and that is accompanied by public education about that strategy. In the absence of effective governance at the federal tier of our government, we did not form a fully federalist strategy but rather generated chaos. It's currently very hard to know what is actually happening in each of the fifty states and eleven territories. The nontransparency of the strategies unfolding in each place is not a sign of successful federalism but rather an indication that we have failed to deploy our federalist structure as the asset it is for harmonized, coordinated, but also modularized and flexible activation of a national strategy.

What makes federalism "federalism" and not chaos is the tie that binds. The national government has the responsibility for forming that tie. Conventionally, for the past century, the president has borne the responsibility for binding our federal structure with national strategy. This White House did not achieve that. Congress might have stepped into the breach, but that branch too failed to meet this responsibility, being riven by a polarized fight over election security throughout the summer and fall months of 2020. There's still a distance to travel to achieve an improved activation of our tiered structure, but one thing that's critical is building knowledge about how it's supposed to work. Our knowledge about the best virtues of our tiered system has atrophied, and that is a major source of our difficulties.

Now some may wonder if the focus on federalism and regionalizing a policy response to a crisis as grave as the COVID-19 pandemic in fact pulls strategy in the wrong direction. After all, is not the pandemic a global problem? Might the relevant governance need be not for devolution but global coordination? The global context is critically important for thinking about this pandemic. Take vaccines as a clear example. Not all countries in the world are able to develop them, yet all are in need of them. We need fair policies for global vaccine distribution, and these do need to be tackled by global bodies. Nonetheless, the regrettable fact is that the absence of civic strength at home—our inability to operate the machinery of our own polity well enough to deliver safety and happiness at home—leaves us ill-equipped to succeed simultaneously at contributing to the broader health of the globe as a whole. Getting our own house in order will be necessary to restoring our ability to be a force for good in the broader world.

4

A Transformed Peace

An Agenda for Healing
Our Social Contract

Before this pandemic hit, we already faced a silent legitimacy crisis. Fewer than 30 percent of people under the age of forty thought that it is essential to live in a democracy. I expect we face a worse legitimacy crisis now.

The pandemic has taught us a dark truth. We don't know, in conditions of emergency, that we will be OK together. Too many people were willing to abandon our elders. As of December 2020, more than 174,000 people had died in America's nursing homes and veterans' facilities (AARP 2020). Too many people were equally willing to abandon essential workers. Those who had to fill essential functions in the early days often worked without personal protective equipment or access to testing. Meatpacking plants and warehouses were rife with outbreaks. Too many people have been willing to abandon the young. Even as it became clear that schools could be opened safely with infection control and ventilation, districts remained committed to remote schooling. Too many people have also been willing to abandon African American and Hispanic/Latinx Americans. Overrepresented in the kinds of service jobs that require in-person interactions, African Americans and Hispanic/Latinx Americans workers by fall 2020 faced unemployment rates twice what they had been before the pandemic hit, even as unemployment rates for the affluent had returned to pre-pandemic levels. Too many people were willing to abandon rural Americans. When we could have kept COVID-19 from reaching rural America, we did not provision rural areas with the tools to spot and suppress outbreaks early and fast. Too many people were willing to limit liberties indefinitely or to act on them abusively. States instituted stay-at-home advisories without end dates while rights activists carried guns into capitol buildings, undermining the health of our social contract.

Hard questions linger. If, in conditions of emergency, we cannot count on support from one another, then how do the institutions we share together have any legitimacy? Why, across this crisis, have too many of us been willing to abandon others among us?

I think the answer to the latter question is fear. Fear for one's own self-preservation has inspired too many to contemplate, openly or secretly, the abandonment of others. Why do we have this fear? We have this fear because we don't have grounds for confidence that, in conditions of emergency, we will be OK together. Why do we not have grounds for confidence? Because even before the pandemic hit, we were not OK together.

In prepandemic conditions of peace, we had already abandoned our elders. Social isolation and loneliness were serious issues for senior citizens even before the pandemic struck (National Institute on Aging 2019).

In prepandemic conditions of peace, we had already abandoned essential workers. The growth of our economy over the last three decades has delivered tremendous material benefits to the best off, while keeping the wages of most workers flat (Mishel et al. 2015).

In prepandemic conditions of peace, we had already abandoned the young. The aging infrastructure of our school buildings, underinvestment in education, and a school-to-prison pipeline for young men of color already meant we were not laying a foundation on which young people could thrive in the future. Our long-standing inability to come to grips with climate change has also meant that older Americans have left younger Americans vulnerable to the existential threat of an inhospitable planet.

In prepandemic conditions of peace, we abandoned black, Hispanic/Latinx, and indigenous Americans. We have watched as overcriminalization, mass incarceration, and violent policing tactics have degraded the health and well-being of communities of color, and we have done relatively little about it, despite having the largest system of penal incarceration in the world.

In prepandemic conditions of peace, we abandoned rural Americans. We watched the nation's economy separate into urban and rural sectors, with rural sectors becoming increasingly distant from opportunity and mobility, and we have not only not delivered solutions but have also largely failed to articulate what they might be.

In prepandemic conditions of peace, we abandoned education about the meaning and value of constitutional democracy and good governance among free and equal citizens. We spent 50 federal dollars per kid each year on STEM education, and only 5 cents on civic education. We have gotten what we paid for.

The pandemic has made visible problems and inequalities that we knew of before the pandemic hit but often put out of our minds. We have long known about inequalities and inequities resulting in worse health outcomes for people of color. Yet the pandemic has given us clarity about the full extent of those disparities.

In that regard, the COVID-19 experience is similar to that of Hurricane Katrina. We knew before Hurricane Katrina hit how unequal New Orleans was, and how broadly unequal Louisiana was. We knew all those things. Yet to see in stark relief just what that meant with regard to mortality and life opportunity was a lesson that the country needed in order to internalize the magnitude of the problem. Moreover, the vulnerability of essential workers and communities of color to COVID-19 has proven to be a vulnerability for all of us. The fact that essential workers have not easily been able to isolate has kept the virus in circulation for everyone. The health inequities are glaring injustices for those who suffer them. Now we can also see that those injustices make us all vulnerable; they weaken us as a society.

How can we develop common purpose, incorporating all of us, and cultivate civic strength when historically marginalized groups within the United States have less ability to make their voices heard, and hence less ability to make sure they're represented within this purpose? In order for anybody to invoke the idea of common purpose with real seriousness, one has to take on the project of healing the social contract. Common purpose has to mean that we're securing well-being for all: happiness and safety for all in the language of the Declaration of Independence. The work of doing that is very much also about paying attention to questions of empowerment in organizations and institutions. We have to rework our political institutions in order to achieve broad empowerment. The question of empowerment—making sure marginalized voices are at decision-making tables—is fundamental to building a healthy social contract and making our world brighter, happier, and more secure for all.

Why should we expect more of ourselves in times of emergency than in times of peace? Frontline health-care workers have brought to this fight a commitment to their fellow residents of this great land that has gone only partially matched by the rest of us. Those health-care workers didn't develop new capacities in a moment of emergency. They took the same standards of care, commitment, and service that shape their daily lives in peace into this crisis.

We yearn for a vision of a future beyond this pandemic. Throughout 2020, one magazine after another asked me to submit a piece sketching what the world would look like "post-pandemic." But I think to ask this question this way was a mistake. This pandemic hasn't changed us or our world. It has simply revealed facts about us to ourselves. It's the old saw: a crisis teaches you who you really are. The world postpandemic will look a lot like our world prepandemic, unless we change who we are.

We were vulnerable as a society to COVID-19 because when it hit, we were not committed to one another or to our constitutional democracy. This disease has spread much more broadly in our society than it would have done if our first instinct society-wide, in response to the first shock of the disease's arrival, had been to marshal the resources necessary to protect the elderly, essential workers, the young, rural Americans whether white, black, indigenous, or Hispanic/Latinx; poor urban Americans whether Hispanic/Latinx, black, indigenous, or white. This disease will spread far wider in our society than it would have done if our go-to instinct with our liberties, in response to the first shock, had been to develop the resources and processes of good governance, and to engage eager defenders of liberty in the question of how we defend our society, lives, livelihoods, and liberties simultaneously.

Our frontline health-care workers took into this pandemic the preexisting peacetime commitments they had to others in our society. The rest of us took into this pandemic our preexisting peacetime commitments to ourselves and our factionalized bonds to personal communities; to self-interest and personal protection rather than a commitment to common purpose.

We won't reach the end of this pandemic and *then* have the chance to develop a transformed peace. If we wish to transform our peace, we will have to effect that transformation during the course of this pandemic. For our preexisting peace is with us still; it defines our response to the virus.

Fear stokes greed, the desire to close the doors and wall out, and to protect whatever "mine" I am currently able to lay my hands on. Greed was already there, but fear makes it worse. How do we exorcise greed?

We all seek safety and happiness, in the words of the Declaration of Independence. If my society can deliver to me a sense of safety, can I relinquish my fear? Will that help me repudiate my greed? Can I see that the only path to safety for any of us in this pandemic is through a broad public project for building safety through disease suppression?

On university campuses with high-powered research facilities—my own included—it was very easy to imagine building and running a program *just for us* that would make it possible for us to open safely. And, in fact, we did build such a program. Similarly, the National Basketball Association learned about this possibility from its connections to universities and built a "bubble" just for itself. But this is like responding to terrorism by encouraging every organization in civil society—whether nonprofit or commercial— to build its own private security corps. Those with resources are protected, everyone else is not. A blameworthy shrug of acceptance on the part of the comfortable sets our course in this direction. The tale of two countries that characterizes our national life—of the affluent and then everyone else—gets worse.

What's the alternative? With terrorism we built a broad public infrastructure of security—ranging from airport security checkpoints to new ways of monitoring public transportation to the ongoing work of people investigating specific threats and networks. Yes, we can see a certain amount of additional private security in our world that has emerged since the events of September 11, 2001. One can't enter many high-rise buildings now without showing identification. But the broad structures of public security mean that everybody is included in the umbrella of protection and uses of private security are minimized. Of course, this is an imperfect example, as the security drive that followed 9/11 also brought with it intense stigmatization of Arab Americans, indeed just as the COVID crisis has generated an increase in hate crimes against Asian Americans. Nonetheless, the underlying point about the need for a public goods approach to COVID response pertains.

We needed a public goods response without stigmatization of others in response to COVID-19. Between March 2020 and the start of 2021, we had enough time to build broad public testing and contact-tracing programs for the whole of our society that would have been able to decelerate and clear out the disease by following chains of transmission, finding every positive case, and supporting people in voluntary isolation. We had the time to build a culture of universal precautions like mask-wearing. Yes, it has been good to have organizations like the University of Chicago, Brown University, and the University of California, San Diego help this public endeavor by contributing resources in support of their communities, but ideally they would have done this as part of a comprehensive and universal infrastructure, not by contributing yet another brick to the ever-growing wall separating the haves from the have-nots.

The idea that we need to rebuild security for all of us through investment in public goods is the best way of capturing what a social contract is. A healthy social contract depends on near universal recognition that there are important goods we all want that we can provision for ourselves much better together than individually. Response to a pandemic is such a public good. The entire point of political institutions—that is, of a social contract consisting of rights and responsibilities—is to deliver public goods of this kind.

Security wards off fear. Escape from fear diminishes the ravening power of greed. It is good to have a release from greed because the republic that will deliver security to me also requires my contribution to it. The republic, or *res publica* in the original Latin—the "public thing"—will improve my life. Does the current crisis caused by coronavirus require a reframing of the balance between public good and individual liberties? No, I don't think so. The goal of securing a constitutional democracy in the face of an existential threat like a pandemic simply is to secure that society *as a constitutional democracy*. In other words, the project of securing the public good, properly understood, is one that fully incorporates the basic liberties. We don't need a rethinking of those fundamental objectives or of how to integrate the idea of the public good and basic liberties. We do need, though, to figure out how to connect our policy decisions to our fundamental overarching objectives. That's where I see the disconnection, not in how we think about public good or think about liberties, but in how we actually activate those commitments at the center of policy deliberation.

How can we rebuild a shared commitment to the public good? We will have to accept smarter and more progressive taxes. Our acceptance of more progressive taxes should flow from our desire to protect our elders, to provide security and opportunity to essential workers, to set the young on a course to exceed their parents in well-being, to include black, Hispanic/Latinx, indigenous, and rural Americans fully in governance, empowerment, and security, to put our liberties to use through practices of good governance.

To accept the need for smarter and more progressive taxes, though, is not to capitulate to statism. We can be smarter about identifying the public goods that need to be delivered through public actors versus those that can be delivered through innovation in the design of market incentives. We need public and private working together, but in both cases with a clear view about the need for a political economy that supports investment in public goods.

We also need to recognize that a sound foundation for health is a right. At the end of the day, one can't legislate for or fully protect people against choices they make that may be detrimental to their health, but everybody should have access to a foundation for health. In the Declaration of Independence's all-important second sentence about self-evident truths, we're introduced to the concept of inalienable rights, but then the text gives us a set of examples, not a complete list. The sentence says, "We hold these truths to be self-evident: that all men are created equal and endowed by their creator with certain inalienable rights, that *among these* are life, liberty and the pursuit of happiness." In other words, we are given three examples of what belongs on that list, not an exhaustive catalog.

I have always read that sentence from the Declaration as a charge to every generation to think through the question of what belongs on *our* list of rights. For our era, I do think a foundation for health belongs there. Our situation differs from the past because of the nature and structure of modern health systems and resources, which are now best provisioned through public good mechanisms. We have to recognize that. To say that, however, is not to answer decisively the question whether there should be private insurance or whether everything should be public; and there are hybrid systems that can deliver a foundation of health for all. But a foundation of health is a right.

Some features of that foundation are newly visible to us thanks to the pandemic. Schools, for instance, are core to how we currently try to provide a foundation for health. This a truth about our social structure that we had previously been unwilling to see. Schools are delivering food, medical care, and sometimes even housing facilities, showers, and the like to children who would otherwise go without. When schools closed to in-person learning, the immediate crisis to be addressed was not a gap in student learning but a more fundamental gap in student access to basic necessities. Schools have accidentally become our welfare infrastructure, something the pandemic has made apparent. Now that we can see where our safety net is, we should strengthen it and give it more capacity and resilience.

We should accept smarter and more progressive taxes to build the public good—structures of safety and happiness that protect all of us together far more effectively than we can achieve if we seek each to do so individually. This does not mean in turn that we abandon our personal responsibility for loving and respecting the specific older people or younger people, or working people, or urban or rural people who are in our immediate networks. To affirm the value of the public good is not to suggest that government should supplant all the good work that civil society does. It is rather to remind us that the good work that we do within our own immediate communities is the seed of an instinct that should be extended, by means of our political institutions, to embrace the whole of our society. If we can reclaim a commitment to a concept of the public good, then we too are lifted up, and given a sturdier foundation for safety and happiness, by the commitment of unnamed others to us, also channeled through our public institutions.

Now if the definition of the pursuit of happiness is something to be rethought in every generation, how do we do that? What constitutes a real conversation about what the pursuit of happiness consists of? Partly we have that conversation already through debates about specific pieces of legislation. We can also have that conversation by working through constitutional amendments. For instance, many citizens are hard at work on a constitutional amendment supporting limits on campaign finance expenditures by corporations. This effort responds to the Supreme Court decision in *Citizens United v. Federal Election Commission* and seeks to restore empowerment to ordinary citizens by reining in the financial power of corporations. Public conversations around pivotal choices like this are occasions for thinking about the pursuit of happiness. How much does genuine empowerment of ordinary people matter to our definition of happiness? That's what is at stake in the effort to undo *Citizens United* through a constitutional amendment.

Of course, we have state constitutions as well as the federal constitution, and amendments to state constitutions show up as ballot propositions in almost every election. We don't pay enough attention to our rights as they are articulated in state constitutions, but there too policy debates give us the opportunity to redefine the pursuit of happiness. For example, there is no right to education in the federal constitution, but there is a right to education in almost every single state constitution. In Rhode Island, a set of plaintiffs is drawing on that state's constitutional right to argue that public education should incorporate preparation for civic life. That's a redefinition of how the state should support the pursuit of happiness.

In the United States social rights—for instance, education and health—are very often attached to and protected in state constitutions rather than in the federal constitution. This is a key feature of the federalist structure I discussed in the last chapter. The centers of gravity for health policy, education policy, and justice policy are all at the state level. Consequently, an effort to rethink the pursuit of happiness in relation to those aspects of life requires engaging at the state level. But of course, as we have seen in the pandemic, the quality of our health infrastructure is not a state question only. It has national implications, including national security implications. As we try to determine which aspects of a given policy area are pertinent locally or regionally, and which aspects are pertinent nationally, and as we seek to harmonize those different aspects, we are constantly renovating and refashioning the frameworks we use to shape and guide the pursuit of happiness.

As with the COVID-19 response, it is the nuts-and-bolts policy conversations that we have that are the vehicle through which our generation will define the pursuit of happiness. When we have these pragmatic policy conversations, it's critical, though, that we actually take time to ask ourselves what values are at stake here. What are our overarching objectives? How do we want to define those overarching objectives? That pivot is necessary to deliver the rich conversation that we can and should have about how we wish to define the pursuit of happiness. It's that pivot—from the practical questions of policy to questions about our overarching values—that doesn't happen often enough, nor with ease and familiarity.

In contemplating a nationwide system of testing, tracing, and supported isolation as the best response to this pandemic, a scientist colleague of mine told me it was doable. He said, "We don't have to break any laws of physics to do it." I've repeated his comment a few times in this book. When he said that to me, I simply nodded in assent. Now I've come to understand the answer I should have given him. "No," I should have said, "we don't have to break the laws of physics. All we have to do is break the laws of politics."

Of course, the laws of politics are not ultimately separable from the laws of physics. Politics happens in time, after all, and what is more fundamental to the laws of physics than time? Politics requires judgment; judgment requires deliberation; deliberation requires conversation and contestation, among parties with widely varying ranges of polarization, competitiveness, or openness to agreement. The more the polarization and competition, the slower the process, and the more time it takes.

The current, highly polarized state of American politics is a physical barrier to successful response to a crisis under time pressure. Democracies always move more slowly than autocracies, even if in the end they can lay down more durable pathways because their choices carry a higher degree of legitimacy and public acceptance. Now, because of our heightened degree of conflict, the temporal dimensions of our politics are moving even more slowly than they might. It has turned out that the laws of our politics could not be broken quickly enough to achieve a national strategy for suppression of COVID-19 that might have kept the disease to low levels. There *were* laws of physics that had to be broken after all—to do with the dynamics of time—they were just packaged as laws of politics.

We may have been more earthbound than we realized in the spring of 2020 when we all craved a solution to our woes. Nonetheless, the lesson persists. To achieve pandemic resilience now and for the future—to achieve justice and health for our constitutional democracy— we will have to break laws of politics. We will have to do this in order to recover our capacity to master time, something fundamentally necessary to handling a crisis. We will have to do this to lay a foundation for a new social contract.

So now in conclusion let me begin the work of breaking some of the laws of politics.

1. Read my lips. We need smarter, more progressive taxes. There are public goods we do need to pay for together.
2. Read my lips. Taxes and the state are not the only answer. We also need innovation so that our market incentives can do a better job of helping private actors function in ways that support public goods.
3. Read my lips. We also need smarter governance. We need elections with real choices; a Congress that works; a Senate with independence from the presidency; and a seat at the decision-making table for people from historically marginalized populations. Accepting smart approaches to

increasing tax revenue should be conditional on reform of our democracy. We shouldn't have to deliver our hard-earned dollars to a broken system. We need to fix our political institutions so that they are worth our investment in them. This was the bargain struck via the Constitution. This is the bargain we need to strike again.

4. Read my lips. We need activists who organize for governance and not just for power. This means organizing to build supermajorities in support of common purpose, not organizing to get to 50 + 1 majorities that can then be wielded as weapons to subdue the other side.

5. Finally, read my lips: we the consumers of contempt-driven media need to stop consuming contempt-driven media. It's on us to make a market for different ways of curating and sharing information and developing usable knowledge.

The starting gun for working on a transformed peace fired at the end of the first quarter of 2020, the point by which the pandemic had already made clear significant vulnerabilities in the state of our existing social contract. If we wish for a transformed peace we must—and better late than never—adopt the following commitments: *We will protect our elders; provide security to essential workers; launch the young; empower and provide a foundation for health to poor rural and urban Americans, whether black, white, or brown; and activate our liberties through support for good governance.* If we can do these things, we will have transformed ourselves, and peace will follow.

Acknowledgments

On March 12, 2020, the day before lockdown started in Massachusetts, I wrote to Ezekiel Emanuel, bioethicist and health policy expert, to ask how an ethics center like ours at Harvard could help address the challenges COVID-19 was presenting our society. We hopped on the phone, and Zeke's answer was that everyone was struggling to figure out how to address what looked like a trade-off between protecting health—by sending everyone into quarantine—and protecting the economy. He thought the intellectual network at our center might be able to help address that question. Thus was born the Edmond J. Safra Center for Ethics's COVID-19 Rapid Response Initiative, to bring rigorous, ethics-centered, multidisciplinary analysis to bear on the crisis. Over the course of the following three months, we published twenty-two white papers (and a final twenty-third in September), two policy road maps, a technical advisory handbook on our TTSI strategy, and several briefings on subjects such as how to achieve pandemic-resilient teaching and learning spaces. We were the first people to put out a bipartisan policy road map arguing for a significant and rapid ramp-up of public investment in testing and contact tracing that laid out how to get it done. Much of our work was ultimately incorporated in the Biden-Harris COVID-19 response, though the dysfunctional politics of our country throughout 2020 meant that our work was only ever applied too little and too late.

Dozens of scholars worked on this effort. We built connections to practitioners at all levels of our government, from Congress and the White House to the National Governors' Association to the National Association of City and County Health Officials to the National Association of State Procurement Officers to specific gubernatorial COVID-19 task forces—and on and on. We reached out to corporate heads and organizations like the Business Roundtable. We reached out to university presidents and organizations like the Association of American Universities and the Council of Independent Colleges. We collaborated with think tanks and policy shops like Vital Strategies, Resolve to Save Lives, New America, the Surgo Foundation, the Breakthrough Institute, Lincoln Labs, and MITRE. Nearly every white paper and all the policy materials were written by teams, their membership sometimes stretching into the dozens. On the core policy road maps we worked hard to build cross-partisan, cross-ideological teams as we hammered our way through tough ethics and policy questions. We had support in this from the Rockefeller Foundation. In the period from March 13 through late May, a core group of us met nightly at 9:15 p.m. The group's composition evolved at that point and those who continued carried on daily at 8:30 a.m. through September, downshifting only then to twice a week, a rhythm we still maintain.

At that May–June pivot point, people were tired, myself included. I paused to look up what a tour of duty on the battlefield had been at earlier points in our history. I learned that in World War II the average tour of duty was six months and in Vietnam it was thirteen months. Given that we were doing our work—as exhausting as it was—by telecommuting from the comfort of our offices, it seemed to me that we had no good excuse to let up only three months in. I chivied everyone on.

This book captures my analysis as it had taken form by June 2020. It was already clear that our politics were dysfunctional and hindering effective COVID-19 response; just how dysfunctional remained yet to be fully seen. Consequently, this book was written from an orientation where success in fighting COVID-19 still seemed imaginable. While the White House had plainly abdicated its responsibility to get the disease under control fast, as of June 2020 it still seemed possible that Congress might act to make the relevant difference. In the end, Congress did not act, having gotten tangled up in a terrible fight over election rules and election integrity.

The work was so intense and the learning from it so profound, as well as personally transformative, that I have chosen to record the learning that emerged out of that most intense period rather than to rewrite this book from the perspective of March 2021, where that backward glance, now also including the Capitol insurrection of January 6 and the murders of Asian Americans in Atlanta, would yield an even gloomier view than presented here.

Thanks go first to the remarkable staff at the Edmond J. Safra Center for Ethics who sprang into action to support the huge body of work we did last spring: Jess Miner, Maggie Gates, Steph Dant, Cherise Fields, Vickie Aldin, Alex Ostrowski-Schilling, and Jake Fay; and to my colleagues on the Safra Faculty Advisory committee who assembled immediately to begin laying the intellectual foundations for our work: especially Arthur Applbaum, Lucas Stanczyk, Mathias Risse, Meira Levinson, Brandon Terry, Tommie Shelby, Bob Truog, David Jones, Glenn Cohen, and Nien-hê Hsieh. Thanks go also to Glen Weyl and Anne-Marie Slaughter for intellectual leadership from start to finish and to Ben Linville-Engler for the same from June when our group evolved. To Lila Tretikov, Meredith Sumpter, and Stefanie Friedhoff for remarkable project coordination and leadership on implementation, on top of intellectual partnership. To Jonathan Hannah, Barbara Smith-Mandell, and Rick Jasculca and Jasculca Terman Associates for jumping in to help us stand up a rapid cottage industry publishing endeavor. To Alicia Bassuk and Eileen O'Connor for having seen the promise in our work and teeing up philanthropic investments to support the effort. To Eric Lander, Matt McKnight, and Andrew Brooks for sharing their depth of expertise about what was technologically possible. (Andrew's death this year from a heart attack is another tragedy stemming, surely, from the intensity of this crisis.) And a final thanks to all the authors on the white papers. May our vision for transformation bear fruit.

References

Allen, Danielle. 2016. "What Is Education for?" *Boston Review*, May 9, 2016. http://bostonreview.net/forum/danielle-allen-what-education.

———. 2020. "A Better Way to Defeat the Virus and Restore the Economy." *Washington Post*, Mar. 26, 2020. https://www.washingtonpost.com/opin ions/2020/03/26/better-way-defeat-virus-restore-economy/.

Allen, Danielle, Sharon Block, et al. 2020. "Roadmap to Pandemic Resilience: Massive Scale Testing, Tracing, and Supported Isolation (TTSI) as the Path to Pandemic Resilience for a Free Society." Edmond J. Safra Center for Ethics COVID-19 Rapid Response Impact Initiative, Apr. 20, 2020. https://ethics.harvard.edu/covid-roadmap.

Allen, Danielle, and Justin Pottle. 2018. "Democratic Knowledge and the Problem of Faction," in Knight Foundation White Paper Series, Trust, Media, and Democracy. https://kf-site-production.s3.amazonaws.com/media _elements/files/000/000/152/original/Topos_KF_White-Paper_Allen_V2 .pdf.

Allen, Danielle, and Emily Sneff. 2019. "Golden Letters: James Wilson, the Declaration of Independence, and the Sussex Declaration." *Georgetown Law Review* 17, no. 1 (Winter 2019), 193–230.

Allen, Danielle, Lucas Stanczyk, et al. 2020. "Securing Justice, Health, and Democracy against the Threat of COVID-19." Edmond J. Safra Center for Ethics COVID-19 Rapid Response Impact Initiative, White Paper no. 1, Mar. 20, 2020. https://ethics.harvard.edu/justice-health-white-paper.

American Association of Retired Persons (AARP), Public Policy Institute. 2020. AARP Nursing Home COVID-19 Dashboard. https://www.aarp .org/ppi/issues/caregiving/info-2020/nursing-home-covid-dashboard .html.

Annenberg Public Policy Center. 2017. "Americans Are Poorly Informed about Basic Constitutional Provisions." Sept. 12, 2017. https://www.anne nbergpublicpolicycenter.org/americans-are-poorly-informed-about-basic -constitutional-provisions/.

Badger, Emily. 2020. "Why an Eviction Ban Alone Won't Prevent a Housing Crisis." *New York Times*, Sept. 3, 2020. https://www.nytimes.com/2020 /09/03/upshot/eviction-moratarium-rent-crisis.html.

Basavaraju, Sridhar V., et al. 2020. "Serologic Testing of U.S. Blood Donations to Identify SARS-CoV-2-reactive Antibodies." *Clinical Infectious Diseases*, Dec. 2019–Jan. 2020, ciaa1785. https://doi.org/10.1093/cid/ciaa1785.

Brandt, Allan, and Alyssa Botelho. 2020. "Not a Perfect Storm—COVID-19 and the Importance of Language." *New England Journal of Medicine* 382: 1493–95. DOI: 10.1056/NEJMp2005032.

Bureau of Economic Analysis. 2020. "Gross Domestic Product, Third Quarter 2020 (Second Estimate." Nov. 25, 2020. https://www.bea.gov/news/2020 /gross-domestic-product-3rd-quarter-2020-second-estimate-corporate -profits-3rd-quarter.

Cammett, Melanie, and Evan Lieberman. 2020. "Building Solidarity: Challenges, Options, and Implications for COVID-19 Responses." Edmond J. Safra Center for Ethics COVID-19 Rapid Response Impact Initiative, White Paper no. 4, Mar. 30, 2020. https://ethics.harvard.edu/building -solidarity.

Centers for Disease Control and Prevention (CDC). 2003. "Use of Quarantine to Prevent Transmission of Severe Acute Respiratory Syndrome—Taiwan, 2003." *Morbidity and Mortality Weekly Report* 52, no. 29 (July 25): 680–83. https://www.jstor.org/stable/23314005.

———. 2004. "Postexposure Prophylaxis, Isolation and Quarantine to Control an Import-Associated Measles Outbreak—Iowa, 2004." *Morbidity and Mortality Weekly Report* 53, no. 41 (Oct. 21): 969–71. https://www.jstor .org/stable/23315472.

———. 2005. "CDC/ASTR Policy on Releasing and Sharing Data." Issued Apr. 16, 2003; updated Sept. 7, 2006. https://www.cdc.gov/maso/policy/releas ingdata.pdf.

———. 2020a. "National Voluntary Accreditation for Public Health Departments." Last updated Apr. 14, 2020. https://www.cdc.gov/publichealth gateway/accreditation/departments.html#LocalHD.

———. 2020b. "COVID-19 Pandemic Planning Scenarios." Sept. 1, 2020. https://www.cdc.gov/coronavirus/2019-ncov/hcp/planning-scenarios .html.

Cohen, Patricia. 2020. "Recession with a Difference: Women Face Special Burden," *New York Times*, Nov. 17, 2020. https://www.nytimes.com/2020/11/17 /business/economy/women-jobs-economy-recession.html.

Conant, Jennet. 2017. *Man of the Hour: James B. Conant, Warrior Scientist.* New York: Simon and Schuster.

DeMuth, Christopher. 2020. "Trump Rewrites the Book on Emergencies." *Wall Street Journal,* Apr. 17, 2020. https://www.wsj.com/articles/trump -rewrites-the-book-on-emergencies-11587142872.

Department of Health and Human Services, Office of the National Coordinator for Health Information Technology. 2014. "Connecting Health and Care for the Nation: A 10-Year Vision to Achieve an Interoperable Health IT Infrastructure." Report released June 2014. https://www.healthit.gov /sites/default/files/ONC10yearInteroperabilityConceptPaper.pdf.

Doerflinger, Thomas, 1986. *A Vigorous Spirit of Enterprise: Merchants and Economic Development in Revolutionary Philadelphia.* Chapel Hill: University of North Carolina Press.

Doi, Asako, Kentaro Iwata, Hirokazu Kuroda, et al. 2020. "Estimation of Seroprevalence of Novel Coronavirus Disease (COVID-19) Using Preserved Serum at an Outpatient Setting in Kobe, Japan: A Cross-Sectional Study." medRxiv 2020.04.26.20079822; DOI: https://doi.org/10.1101/2020 .04.26.20079822.

Emanuel, Ezekiel J., Susan Ellenberg, and Michael Levy. 2020. "The Coronavirus Is Here to Stay, so What Happens Next?" *New York Times,* Mar. 17, 2020. https://www.nytimes.com/2020/03/17/opinion/coronavirus-social-dis tancing-effect.html.

Eilperin, Juliet, Laurie McGinley, Steven Mufson, and Josh Dawsey, 2020. "In the Absence of a National Testing Strategy, States Go Their Own Way." *Washington Post,* Apr. 8, 2020. https://www.washingtonpost.com/health /2020/04/07/testing-coronavirus-trump/.

Fallows, Deborah. 2020. "A Rural Health Center with a Pandemic Plan." *Atlantic,* Apr. 9, 2020. https://www.theatlantic.com/notes/2020/04/little -town-pandemic-plan/609715/.

Federalist Papers. Avalon Project of the Lillian Goldman Law Library at Yale Law School. https://avalon.law.yale.edu/subject_menus/fed.asp.

Ferguson, Neil M., Daniel Laydon, Gemma Nedjati-Gilani, et al. 2020. "Impact of Non-pharmaceutical Interventions (NPIs) to Reduce COVID-19 Mortality and Healthcare Demand." Imperial College COVID-19 Response Team, Report 9, Mar. 16, 2020. https://spiral.imperial.ac.uk:8443/handle /10044/1/77482.

Finnemore, Martha, and Michelle Jurkovich, "The Politics of Aspiration." *International Studies Quarterly (ISQ),* June 28, 2020. https://doi.org/10.1093 /isq/sqaa052; available at SSRN: https://ssrn.com/abstract=3637566.

Flaxman, Seth, Swapnil Mishra, Axel Gandy, et al. 2020. "Estimating the Number of Infections and the Impact of Non-pharmaceutical Interventions on COVID-19 in 11 European Countries." Imperial College COVID-19 Response Team, Report 13, Mar. 30, 2020. https://www.imperial.ac.uk /media/imperial-college/medicine/mrc-gida/2020-03-30-COVID19 -Report-13.pdf.

Foa, Roberto Stefan, and Yascha Mounk. 2016. "The Danger of Deconsolidation: The Democratic Disconnect." *Journal of Democracy* 27, no. 3 (July): 5–17.

Fussell, Chris, Jennifer Keister, and Keith Pelligrini. 2020. "Fusion Cell Playbook." McChrystal Group, posted Apr. 14, 2020. https://www.linkedin.com /feed/update/urn:li:activity:6655838457199493120/.

Garde, Damian, and Jonathan Saltzman. 2020. "The Story of mRNA: How a Once-Dismissed Idea Became a Leading Technology in the Covid Vaccine Race." *STAT*, Nov. 10, 2020. https://www.statnews.com/2020/11/10/the-story -of-mrna-how-a-once-dismissed-idea-became-a-leading-technology-in-the -covid-vaccine-race/.

Gerken, Heather K. 2020. "Second-Order Diversity: An Exploration of Decentralization's Egalitarian Possibilities." In *Diversity, Justice, and Democracy*, ed. Danielle Allen and Rohini Somanathan, 227–62. Chicago: University of Chicago Press.

Gostin, Lawrence, James G. Hodge, and Lindsay F. Wiley. 2020. "Presidential Powers and Response to COVID-19." *Journal of the American Medical Association* 323, no. 16 (April 28): 1547–48.

Government Accountability Office (GAO). 2020. "COVID-19: Urgent Actions Needed to Better Ensure an Effective Federal Response." Nov. 30, 2020. https://www.gao.gov/products/gao-21-191.

Haberman, Maggie, and David E. Sanger. 2020. "Trump Says Coronavirus Cure Cannot 'Be Worse Than the Problem Itself.'" *New York Times*, Mar. 23, 2020. https://www.nytimes.com/2020/03/23/us/politics/trump-coronavirus-re strictions.html.

Hansmann, Lisa, and Ganesh Sitaraman. 2020. "Interstate Compacts: A Primer." Edmond J. Safra Center COVID-19 Rapid Response Impact Initiative, White Paper no. 13, Apr. 30, 2020. https://ethics.harvard.edu/files /center-for-ethics/files/interstatecompactsprimer.pdf.

Horgan, John. 2020. "Will COVID-19 Make US Less Democratic and More like China? The Pandemic Has Revealed the Disadvantages of Laissez-Faire Governance and Advantages of Centralized Control." *Scientific American*, Apr. 27, 2020. https://blogs.scientificamerican.com/cross-check/will -covid-19-make-us-less-democratic-and-more-like-china/.

Jha, Ashish, and Sameer Nair-Desai. 2020. "The Case for Open Schools in a Pandemic." *Pandemics Explained*, Nov. 16, 2020. https://globalepidemics .org/2020/11/16/the-case-for-open-schools-in-a-pandemic/.

Jha, Ashish, Thomas Tsai, and Benjamin Jacobson. 2020. "Why We Need at Least 500,000 Tests per Day to Open the Economy—and Stay Open." Harvard Global Health Institute, posted Apr. 17, 2020. https://globalepi demics.org/2020/04/18/why-we-need-500000-tests-per-day-to-open-the -economy-and-stay-open/.

Johnstone-Louis, Mary, Bridget Kustin, Colin Mayer, Judith Stroehle, and Boya Wang. 2020. "Business in Times of Crisis," *Oxford Review of Economic Policy* 36, no. S1: S242–55.

Jones, David, and Meredith Rosenthal. 2020. "Preparedness and Unpreparedness: The Military vs. Medicine." Edmond J. Safra Center COVID-19 Rapid Response Impact Initiative, White Paper no. 15, May 7, 2020. https:// ethics.harvard.edu/files/center-for-ethics/files/15militarymedicine.pdf.

Laughland, Oliver, and Amanda Holpuch. 2020. "'We're Modern Slaves': How Meat Plant Workers Became the New Frontline in COVID-19 War." *Guardian*, May 2, 2020. https://www.theguardian.com/world/2020/may/02/meat -plant-workers-us-coronavirus-war.

Leprince-Ringuet, Daphne. 2020. "Contact Tracing: Data Shows Apps Can Help in Fight against COVID, Say Researchers: The Team behind Switzerland's SwissCovid App Have Shown Promising Results for the Tool." *ZDNet*, Sept. 7, 2020. https://www.zdnet.com/article/contact-tracing-data -shows-apps-can-help-in-fight-against-covid-say-researchers/.

Levinson, Meira, and Jacob Fay. 2020. "Educational Ethics During a Pandemic." Edmond J. Safra Center for Ethics COVID-19 Rapid Response Impact Initiative, White Paper no. 17, May 16, 2020. https://ethics.har vard.edu/files/center-for-ethics/files/17educationalethics2.pdf.

Marcus, David. 2020. "Trump's Federalist Approach to the Virus Is Working." *Federalist*, May 8, 2020. https://thefederalist.com/2020/05/08/trumps -federalist-approach-to-the-virus-is-working/.

McCarthy, Justin. 2018. "Americans Still More Trusting of Local than State Government." Gallup, Oct. 8, 2018. https://news.gallup.com/poll/243563 /americans-trusting-local-state-government.aspx.

McDowall, Angus, and Ayat Basma. 2017. "Middle East Wars Forcing Change in Approach to Medical Care: Extra Patients and Collapsed Systems Amplify Problems." *Scientific American*, May 16, 2017. https://www.scientificamer ican.com/article/middle-east-wars-forcing-change-in-approach-to-med ical-care/.

McKillop, Matt, and Vinu Ilakkuvan. 2019. "The Impact of Chronic Underfunding on America's Public Health System: Trends, Risks, and Recommendations, 2019." Trust for America's Health, n.d. https://www.tfah.org /wp-content/uploads/2020/03/TFAH_2019_PublicHealthFunding_07 .pdf.

Mishel, Lawrence, Elise Gould, and Josh Bivens. 2015. "Wage Stagnation in Nine Charts." Economic Policy Institute, Jan. 6, 2015. https://www.epi.org/publication/charting-wage-stagnation/.

Moktar, Faris. 2020. "How Singapore Flipped from Virus Hero to Cautionary Tale." *Bloomberg*, Apr. 21, 2020. https://www.bloomberg.com/news/articles/2020-04-21/how-singapore-flipped-from-virus-hero-to-cautionary-tale.

Moore, Dasia. 2020. "Across the State, Lengthy Lines for COVID-19 Testing Reflect a Bigger Problem." *Boston Globe*, Nov. 27, 2020. https://www.bostonglobe.com/2020/11/27/nation/across-state-long-lines-covid-19-testing-reflect-bigger-problem/?p1=SectionFront_Feed_ContentQuery.

National Academy of Sciences, National Academy of Engineering, and Institute of Medicine. 2007. *Rising above the Gathering Storm: Energizing and Employing America for a Brighter Economic Future*. Washington, DC: National Academies Press.

National Commission on Excellence in Education. US Department of Education. 1983. *A Nation at Risk: The Imperative for Educational Reform*. https://www2.ed.gov/pubs/NatAtRisk/risk.html.

National Conference of State Legislatures. 2017. "Drug Testing for Welfare Recipients and Public Assistance." Mar. 24, 2017. https://www.ncsl.org/research/human-services/drug-testing-and-public-assistance.aspx.

National Institute on Aging. 2019. "Social Isolation, Loneliness in Older People Pose Health Risks." Apr. 23, 2019. https://www.nia.nih.gov/news/social-isolation-loneliness-older-people-pose-health-risks.

Pelosi, Nancy. 2019. "Floor Speech in Support of Resolution for Open Hearings on Trump's Abuse of Power." Oct. 31, 2019. https://www.speaker.gov/newsroom/103119.

Pew Research Center. 2017. "The Partisan Divide on Political Values grows Even Wider." Oct. 5, 2017. https://www.pewresearch.org/politics/2017/10/05/1-partisan-divides-over-political-values-widen/.

Pew Research Center. 2019. "Public Trust in Government: 1958–2019." Apr. 11, 2019. https://www.people-press.org/2019/04/11/public-trust-in-government-1958-2019/.

Prevent Epidemics. 2020. "Adaptive Reponse." April 1, 2020. https://preventepidemics.org/covid19/science/insights/adaptive-response/.

Public Health Leadership Society (PHLS). 2002. "Principles of the Ethical Practice of Public Health." Version 2.2. https://www.apha.org/-/media/files/pdf/membergroups/ethics/ethics_brochure.ashx.

Reynolds, D. L., J. R. Garay, S. L. Deamond, et al. 2008. "Understanding Compliance and Psychological Impact of the SARS Quarantine Experience." *Epidemiology and Infection* 136, no. 7 (July): 997–1007.

Rivers, Caitlin, Christina Silcox, Christina Potter, et al. 2020. "Risk Assessment and Testing Protocols for Reducing SARS-CoV-2 Transmission in K-12 Schools." Duke-Margolis Center for Health Policy. https://healthpol icy.duke.edu/sites/default/files/2020-10/Risk%20Assessment%20and%20 Testing%20Protocols%20for%20Reducing%20SARS-CoV-2%20Transmis sion%20in%20K-12%20Schools_14%20Oct%202020.pdf.

Rockefeller Foundation. 2020. "National Covid-19 Testing Action Plan: Pragmatic Steps to Reopen Our Workplaces." Rockefeller Foundation, Apr. 21, 2020. https://www.rockefellerfoundation.org/wp-content/uploads/2020/04 /TheRockefellerFoundation_WhitePaper_Covid19_4_22_2020.pdf.

Rucker, Philip, and William Wan. 2020. "Trump Projects Up to 240,000 Coronavirus Deaths in U.S., Even with Mitigation Efforts." *Washington Post*, Mar. 30, 2020. https://www.washingtonpost.com/politics/trump -white-house-projects-up-to-240000-coronavirus-deaths-in-us-even-with -mitigation-efforts/2020/03/31/62df5344-7367-11ea-87da-77a8136c1a6d _story.html.

Schaart, Eline, Lili Bayer, and Katie Jennings. 2019. "Finland's Government Collapses over Failed Health Care Reform: PM Juha Sipilä Resigns." *Politico*, Mar. 8, 2019. https://www.politico.eu/article/finlands-government-collapses -over-failed-health-care-reform/.

Secon, Holly, and Aylin Woodward. 2020. "About 95% of Americans Have Been Ordered to Stay at Home. This Map Shows Which Cities and States Are Under Lockdown." *Business Insider*, Apr. 7, 2020. https://www.busi nessinsider.com/us-map-stay-at-home-orders-lockdowns-2020-3.

Sethi, Rajiv, Divya Siddarth, Nia Johnson, et al. 2020. "Who Is Dying and Why?" Edmond J. Safra Center for Ethics COVID-19 Rapid Response Impact Initiative, White Paper no. 19, May 20, 2020. https://ethics.har vard.edu/files/center-for-ethics/files/19cwhoisdying.pdf.

Smith, Charles Page. 1956. *James Wilson, Founding Father, 1742–1798*. Chapel Hill: University of North Carolina Press.

Watson, Crystal, Anita Cicero, James Blumenstock, et al. 2020. "A National Plan to Enable Comprehensive COVID-19 Case Finding and Contact Tracing in the US." Johns Hopkins, Bloomberg School of Public Health, Center for Health Security, Apr. 10, 2020. https://www.centerforhealthsecurity .org/our-work/pubs_archive/pubs-pdfs/2020/a-national-plan-to-enable -comprehensive-COVID-19-case-finding-and-contact-tracing-in-the-US .pdf.

Weyl, Glen, et al. 2020. "Mobilizing the Political Economy for COVID-19." Edmund J. Safra Center for Ethics, Harvard University, White Paper no. 3, Mar. 26, 2020. https://drive.google.com/file/d/17kGMznpxIuUPdP3 icqXkxIsqqQ0sTtY7/view.

Whalen, Jeanne, Tony Romm, Aaron Gregg, and Tom Hamburger. 2020. "Scramble for Medical Equipment Descends into Chaos as U.S. States and Hospitals Compete for Rare Supplies." *Washington Post*, Mar. 24, 2020. https://www.washingtonpost.com/business/2020/03/24/scramble -medical-equipment-descends-into-chaos-us-states-hospitals-compete -rare-supplies/.

Williams, David, Sarah Oppenheimer, Danielle Allen, and Meredith Sumpter. 2020. "The Economic Case for Robust Public Health Intervention to Stop COVID." *Pandemics Explained*, Oct. 14, 2020. https://globalepidemics.org /2020/10/14/the-economic-case-for-robust-public-health-intervention -to-stop-covid/.

World Health Organization (WHO). 2009. "Analysing Disrupted Health Sectors: A Modular Manual." https://www.who.int/hac/techguidance/tools /disrupted_sectors/adhsm.pdf.

———. 2020. "COVID-19 Weekly Epidemiological Update." Dec. 22, 2020. https://www.who.int/docs/default-source/coronaviruse/situation-reports /20201222_weekly_epi_update_19.pdf.

Wylie, Melissa. 2018. "Surprising Stats on Drugs in the Workplace." *Biz- women*, Jan. 18, 2018. https://www.bizjournals.com/bizwomen/news/latest -news/2018/01/surprising-stats-on-drugs-in-the-workplace.html.

Yang, Yuan, and Nian Liu, Sue-Lin Wong, and Qianer Liu. 2020. "China, Coronavirus and Surveillance: The Messy Reality of Personal Data." *Financial Times*, Apr. 2, 2020. https://www.ft.com/content/760142e6-740e-11ea-95fe -fcd274e920ca.

Index

Note: Page numbers in italics refer to figures or tables.